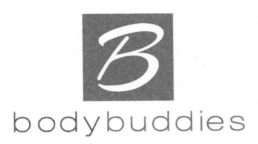

The Power Foods Lifestyle

Kristy Jo Hunt, CPT/FNS
Founder/CEO, *Body Buddies*

Published by Ringmasters

To all of my Body Buds near and far,

I admire you for your great undertaking to turn obstacles and adversity into victory and self-mastery. You are my inspiration and the very reason I seek to reach out and help.
This book is dedicated to you.

Love your bud,

Kristy Jo

What Body Buddies are saying about *The Power Foods Lifestyle*™

"Great book! It is very easy reading and easy to understand. Never question again which Power Foods will help you get to your goal!"
—*Sandee Davis*

"My husband and I have enjoyed eating healthily for many years, but we have not been able to reach our final goals. It seemed that we just needed something more but did not know where to turn. When we read The Power Foods Lifestyle together we were able to see what we were doing wrong and what we were missing. With a little preparation every day we started eating better than before and we were able to reach our goals. Now we have a lifestyle that works so well for us and our family."
—*Josh and Cambria Penrod*

"I am so glad I found Body Buddies. Not only do I feel better than I ever have, but I feel like I finally understand my body. Strange I know, that it has taken 34 years to figure it out, but better late than never. I have lost 10% body fat, gained a good deal of muscle, and I have saved quite a bit of money because I am not eating out all the time. Thank you so much!"
—*Monti Warren-Bargsley*

"I have become more disciplined in every aspect of my life at work spiritually and in the confidence I have in myself. I have learned how to choose foods based on how my body will feel in the future, rather than getting that immediate pleasure out of a sugary treat."
—*Trent Tippetts*

"The Power Foods Lifestyle is life changing! It tells you what kind of food to eat and how often to eat. It takes the guesswork out of eating healthy and balanced meals. Power Foods keep you energized throughout the day and feeling amazing!! I haven't felt this great about myself and my health in years, even after having two kids! Thanks for answering my prayers."
—*Michelle Fox*

"Great book! It's very easy to read and understand and a great foundation for eating better for life! I love this book and the empowerment it has given me coupled with hiring Kristy Jo as a nutrition coach. I am now trained on living and eating the Power Foods my body craves! I have more energy and am much healthier living the Power Foods Lifestyle!"
—*Stephanie Schmid*

"I have developed new eating habits. I can't believe that I eat carrots in the morning! And I eat so many more vegetables than I used to. I used to be very dependent on carbs, but now I don't even miss them in my PVF meals. I eat way more protein now that I used to. I feel like these are habits and routines I have learned to love and do without effort, so I know I have made a lifestyle change, not just a diet change. I have learned how to separate fat and carbs! It's not hard to do once you figure out some meals to eat. I'm just used to it now and it all still tastes good and now when I do have fat and carbs, it feels like a real treat. Pairing a veggie with everything makes me feel more full and have more energy throughout the day."
—*Michelle Larsen*

"I have learned so much about nutrition. I didn't realize how eating the "right" foods can really make my body feel good. I almost never have headaches anymore. Just this one change has made me a believer in the PFL lifestyle. I also lost some weight, so that was a really good motivator too."
—*Rachel Newman*

Your habits are a result of your thought patterns.

We will begin by focusing on your mind.

You will learn how to discipline yourself.

The changes you make will be permanent.

The Power Foods Lifestyle will become *your* lifestyle.

The strategies of this lifestyle will guide you to improved health and confidence.

You will become the master of yourself.

The Power Foods Lifestyle

About the Author and Body Buddies

I'm a bit of a random person. I like to play with my Nerf gun. I speak near-fluent Korean. Peanut butter and jelly sandwiches are my indulgence—I could eat them all day long. I've tickled the ivories since I was eight. Reading the dictionary is my guilty pleasure. I'm pretty much just a nerd with a very intense passion for nutrition, fitness, and helping the people around me learn to feel confident and happy in their own skin. I am also a Certified Personal Trainer, Fitness Nutrition Specialist, dance judge and choreographer, and coach to a natural bodybuilding team.

I'm Kristy Jo and Body Buddies is my creation. As your Bud, I hope to inspire and motivate you on a daily basis. I accomplish this primarily through the Body Buddies Podcast, Facebook page and Instagram feed. I hope that daily visits to these free socialmedia platforms will inspire and teach you to live a healthy lifestyle, keeping you fired up to reach your goals. You can find them at the URLs below:

"Body Buddies" Podcast – iTunes and Stitcher Radio app
www.facebook.com/bodbuds
www.instagram.com/bodbuds

I do my best to disseminate the overload of information out there and re-package it in a way that you can understand and apply. I teach through Facebook, YouTube, Instagram, Podcast, and my weekly emails. I do my best to provide a lot of FREE information, in addition to providing custom coaching opportunities by my team of incredible Body Buddies® coaches. You may learn more about these services as you continue investigating this way of life by heading over to my site:

www.body-buddies.com

As the fourth of seven children, I've gained a great appreciation for family and relationships. People are the most important part of this life. It didn't take me long to realize the more I serve others, the happier I become and the more purpose my life has. This is why I love running Body Buddies. It's such an honor to be able to provide information to help people like you live a healthier and happier life.

I find that self-disclosure is what brings people closer. I'd like you to feel that you know and trust me, and so I'd like to share a little (and maybe more than a little) about myself:

I began dancing when I was twelve. From the first day I walked into a studio, dance was my life and every breath. I studied jazz, ballet, hip hop, modern, contemporary and ballroom. After years of dancing as a member of my studio's competition team, high school drill team, competing in numerous individual competitions, coaching my high school team after graduating, teaching dance in private studios, judging competitions, teaching workshops and choreography, and dancing on the Dixie State University dance company, I was accepted to the MFA program (Masters of Fine Arts) modern dance program at the University of Utah. I was thrilled to be pursuing my dream of becoming an artistic director of dance for a university.

However, the serious back pain that intensified during heavy rehearsals and performances scared me. My senior year of college revolved around dealing with the ever-increasing agony. When it became too much for me to handle on my own, I forced myself into a doctor's office. Prior to the visit, I knew I had scoliosis. I had known this from the time I was fifteen years old and become immobile due to landing incorrectly at dance rehearsal. A visit to the chiropractor and a few x-rays later, my lateral scoliosis (where the spine curves like an 'S') was revealed. Fortunately, I'd suffered very little pain up until then—only mild muscular fatigue after too much time on my feet. Until my late college years, the misalignment had given me incredible flexibility that enhanced my abilities as a dancer.

After two orthopedic surgeons cautioned me to halt my dancing, advising that I put a rod in my back to straighten my spine, I began to consider my life and how all of my dancing dreams would never come to fruition. Motivated by the desire to fix this great obstacle, I buried myself in heavy research, after which

I decided that I would not have surgery. After much contemplation and prayer, I decided I would rather have a shorter but higher quality life than a longer life of lesser quality. That was my decision then, and still to this day, I know that was the right decision for me.

With consistent chiropractic care (thanks to Dr. Shetlin at South Jordan Chiropractic who cared for my spine both in St. George, Utah and currently in Salt Lake City, Utah) and rigorous nutrition and fitness habits, my orthopedic doctors are changing their minds about my condition. In 2011, they told me I would be in a wheelchair by age 40 and that my spine would begin to move into the region where my lungs are by age 60, which could possibly end my life. In 2013, they told me that by staying active and eating well I may be able to keep myself out of a wheelchair—permanently. As a result of my habits, the curvature of my spine has actually decreased and regular chiropractic care is keeping arthritis from setting in. In 2015, at the time of the revision of this book, the curve remains stable thanks to the muscle I have built. Proper stretching and training each day are critical to my mobility, and it's paramount I use variations of traditional weight lifting movements in order to protect my back. Living with chronic pain gives me empathy for others, and gratitude for all the things I am able to do. Being able to walk each day is a gift on its own. Everything in addition to that is a cherry on top.

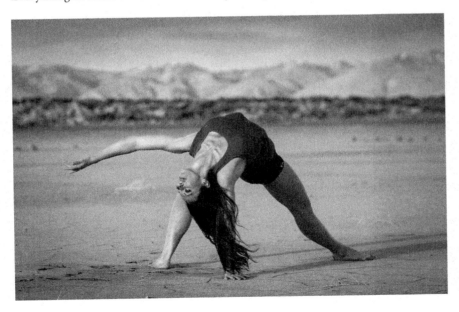

Though in 2011 I left behind my dream of becoming an artistic dance director, the disordered eating habits and thoughts that plagued me from the time I was nine years old remained.

For nearly 15 years, I struggled with obsessive calorie-counting and restrictive diets in efforts to lose weight. After a time of dieting intensely, my resolve broke, resulting in horrific binge-eating episodes of anywhere from 5,000-10,000 calories in a single sitting. In order to punish myself for the behavior and prevent the weight gain I feared, I forced myself to vomit immediately following the binge and spend hours at the gym to burn as many calories as possible. I exercised so viciously that I often developed injuries. Even still, I forced myself to continue exercising. Voices of disdain, loathing, anger, and disgust constantly screamed in my mind. I hated myself and I hated that no matter how hard I tried, I could not break my obsessive cycle of behavior. I felt alone and that no one could ever help me.

My family, friends, academic and dance peers, as well as co-workers all knew me as a health nut—what they didn't see was the dark side of me I kept private and hidden from the world. I was ashamed of who I was in secret, and put that much more effort into a happy and bubbly public appearance. I didn't want anyone to know my burdens.

When I was 25, I'd finally had enough. I decided that I could not and would not continue living life the way I had. I hated myself. I ridiculed myself. I loathed myself. 15 years of this was enough. I wanted discipline. I wanted control. I wanted to be the master of my habits and behavior.

On March 17, 2012, something inside of me snapped. Many things in my life weren't going right—I was failing in my dating relationships, liked my job and had an amazing boss, yet didn't feel I was achieving all I had the potential to do in a career, and felt miserable with my body and spirituality. Driving home that afternoon from a weekend getaway at a friend's house, I felt a thought swell inside my head so large that I felt it expand like a balloon.

You are the master of yourself.

The phrase repeated itself over and over in my mind. Caught off guard, I lifted my hand to adjust the rear-view mirror until I was looking at my reflection. I stared myself down. Did that really come from me? I thought. No matter if the voice was a product of my subconscious or a message from a loving and eternal God, the thought was real, and it lodged deep inside me. In that moment, I knew that I could shape my own life and would do so from that day forward; I would prove to myself that I could do anything—and I would begin with my body. If I could discipline my body and my mind, I knew the rest of my life would fall into place.

For the first time, I followed through with a goal to completely change my body. It was the most grueling process I've ever experienced, but I transformed my body, my mind, and my entire life in a short eight weeks. I competed in three Women's Figure competitions (a category of women's bodybuilding) that summer, placing in the top three at each event.

I finished the season at 11% body fat, but knew that I couldn't maintain such a low level and still be healthy. The competition diet I had been following was too restrictive and extreme to maintain. Additionally, my doctor had become concerned with my blood labs—my liver was showing elevated AST and ALT numbers. I went to work researching how to maintain a healthy 16-17% body fat level.

The Power Foods Lifestyle™ is a product of my disciplined experimentation—trials and errors alike— to maintain my competition lean body in the healthiest way possible. I had heard so much about competitors going "psycho" after their disciplined "dieting down" and then gaining deplorable amounts of weight once they were "free." I didn't want to be one of them! Additionally, I had heard about all of this metabolic damage and insulin resistance that competition diets created. Again, I didn't want to deal with that! I wanted truth and I knew it had to be out there. As I slowly discovered what worked for my body, I began sharing my findings with friends and family. I was surprised to see that this way of eating helped those close to me to feel better, healthier, more energetic, and ultimately lose body fat.

I realized that more people needed to hear what I'd discovered. I began sharing the principles more openly through the Facebook page I had created called Body Buddies, even though I was nervous that I would be ridiculed by dietitians for teaching people how to eat without a state license. As such, I built upon the qualifications I'd earned when I'd received my Personal Training certification in 2010 by becoming a certified Fitness Nutrition Specialist through the National Academy of Sports Medicine.

The Power Foods method of eating is a simple summary of all of the nutritional and food chemistry research I came upon and how this science relates to sculpting the body. While the research and evidence fascinates me, I know that the general population could care less. I strive to separate fact from fiction when it comes to nutrition and exercise, and summarize ideas and strategies in ways that are easy for you to understand and apply to your life. I hope to someday receive an email from you telling me about how you have started transforming your body and your mind—and how good you feel! When this happens, you can reach me at kristyjo@ body-buddies.com.

At the time of the revision of this book in 2015, I have coached over 1,000 people through the process of living this lifestyle, seen incredible transformations, shed many tears of happiness, and watched as one small drop of hope for myself has had incredible ripple effects of change for so many people. It's extremely humbling to watch this all happen. Now, with my team of coaches, I'm able to reach more and more people. I hope that you will read this book and my philosophy with an open mind and an intent to understand principles, not to a search for a magical diet.

I don't claim to know everything, but I'm constantly engaged in research and attending nutrition and exercise seminars to learn more. The health industry is full of lots of quacks, bogus ideas, and strategies simply to expand profit margins. I feel it's my duty to sift through the vast information to find the most practical and strategic method for each of my clients and all in this ever-growing family of Body Buddies. I hope you will take advantage of the Body Buddies Family communities (like joining the private group Power Foods Lifestyle Champions on Facebook) and seek to help others around you, too. We can't all change the world, but we can help one person at a time.

1

A Healthy Lifestyle is Maintainable

Welcome to the world of Body Buddies and your introduction to the Power Foods Lifestyle. I'm so glad you're here! I think it's safe to assume that you are reading this book because you want to succeed at changing your body and your mind. You want to lose fat, tone, or even build muscle, be healthy, and feel in control of yourself. You want to feel like your clothes fit you well. You want to feel confident in a swim suit. You want to feel energetic and positive about life. You want to better cope with, or prevent, chronic illness. You're ready for change.

I want you to know that you can do this. You really can. It all begins with the desire to learn, then try, then continue trying. That effort will turn into results. I promise you there's a person inside you who's stronger than any obstacle you'll face.

You're about to find that person.

But it's going to take some work, and we both know that.

Why We Are the Way We Are

The health industry doesn't make it easy to lose weight and get healthy. They overwhelm you with diets that promise you'll drop weight in no time flat with little effort. Thanks to the Internet, bookstores, and magazines, the information—and misinformation—at your fingertips is virtually unlimited.

I know firsthand how easy it is to become overwhelmed by so many different theories, recommendations and products. I've swung from diet to diet and from promise to promise like you may have, all in hopes of finding the one method out there that would give me the results I wanted.

Meanwhile, unhealthy, yet incredibly tempting foods are marketed to you through television, radio, social media, and billboards. Over the years, these food-like substances have become a normal way of life and society as a whole has come to accept them as commonplace. Eating processed and packaged foods seems to be the norm—the American way of life. That is how we cope with chaotic schedules, endless lists of to-dos, and our ongoing emotional battles.

Traditional behavior has resulted in society not even thinking about the harm they're doing to their bodies. Add this lack of awareness to the nearly unmanageable stress levels we all experience, and food becomes an escape, a reward, and a relief. When experiencing stress and difficult life circumstances, not just any food will do—only delicious and convenient food seems to provide respite. No wonder over 69% of Americans over the age of 20 are overweight or obese.

Thanks to the common lifestyle—as well as the over-publicized images of models, fitness junkies, and athletes—I've come to learn that most people feel negative emotions about their appearance. It can be easy to feel even worse about yourself if you know that something is lacking in your life in terms of discipline and control. You may even justify the way you look and feel because you don't want to be accused of being "obsessed" about your appearance and health. And so the behaviors continue, and the lack of discipline and accepting reality begins to manifest itself physically in your shape, possibly even in the form of disease or life-threatening illness.

Stop the Desperation Diets

Are you someone that has found yourself so desperate to "fix" your weight that you felt something needed to be done quickly? Have you turned to the latest fad diet or crazed exercise plan in hopes that it held the answer to your desperation—to fix your waistline, your risk for disease, or your emotional fluctuations? Have you learned that nearly every fad diet is impossible to maintain in the long-term? Sure, these diets may deliver results in eight to twelve weeks, but will those changes be permanent? No—because these focus on fixing only your body, not on what we are going to work on together: improving your behavior, *which is a direct result of the strength of your mind.*

When a dieter loses his or her determination and willpower to follow the diet, he or she returns—usually in excess—to former habits. Once again, can you relate? I sure can! I've tried about every single diet out there, and failed miserably at each one. Sure, I did great for a few days, and even sometimes a few weeks, but inevitably my willpower broke and I ended up back in my binging cycles. I ate like a crazed hyena that had been starved to kingdom come! Then, plagued by guilt, I turned to vomiting or excessive exercise to eliminate my crazed feasting. It breaks my heart to remember how miserable I felt and the self-loathing that plagued me from the ages of nine to twenty-five. I hope that no one else ever has to experience those difficult emotions. Unfortunately, I know they are very commonplace.

The dieting needs to stop. Nearly every diet or quick-weight-loss plan I've come across is unhealthy for long-term maintenance. These diets and plans recommend an imbalanced ratio of macronutrients (protein, carbohydrates, and fat—to be discussed in a later chapter) or eliminate entire food groups completely. All types of naturally-occurring foods play a role in our health and should never be cut out entirely. Instead, they should be understood, respected, and used strategically. That is what the Power Foods Lifestyle is all about: strategy.

Good thing you're here. You can now find the confidence and joy of knowing that you're going to learn the strategic and healthy way to change your mind, body, and habits. This means it's not going to be overnight, but it's going to be the true change in outlook and behavior you need to maintain it. In order to begin to understand yourself, a little introspection and thinking about who you are and how you feel is required.

Introspection Time

Let's chat about your body and how you view it. I'd like you to take a moment to ponder and jot down a few notes. Please don't skip this section—it's an important exercise for you to do. Grab a pen or pencil and fill in the blanks with your current emotions and thoughts before moving on:

My body is _____.

Others view my body as _____.

I wish my body _____.

Alright, put your pen or pencil down and let's talk about what you wrote.

- What are the words that are in the blanks?
- Are they negative words?
- Are they positive words?
- Does this show you more about how you view your body?
- Do you look at your body as a blessing or a curse?

No matter what you wrote down, we are going to work on improving the way you view your body. The vehicle of your body is how you experience your life—it's a blessing and not something to be hated or despised. It's something for which to be grateful and treat with respect. I know you may not agree with me right now, but I'd like you to really try to think in this new plane.

What are you able to do? Are you able to walk? Breathe? Smile? Do you have at least one person who loves you? Are you able to see? Hear? I have dear friends without legs, hearing capabilities, or vision—and they are some of the happiest people I know! Gratitude is one of the key values that we need to begin integrating into the way you think. When you are grateful for what you have, instead of what you don't have, you will begin to experience a new kind of life.

No way is life easy! There is much that happens that could make you angry and bitter. It's very easy to compare your life to others and feel like, somehow, somewhere, you got shafted. Social media certainly doesn't help this cause, and you can become entrapped in the constant comparison game which you will never win. There will always be someone fitter, younger, richer, and smarter than you. So what? Should that take away from the wonder and joy of you and your life?

Though it may not seem like it, every single person is tried, tested, and pummeled with difficulties in many ways—not just you. Curveballs that throw everyone off seem to come regularly. We can hardly predict what will come our way next.

For many people, their body and the way they feel about it is one of the greatest challenges in their lives. Whether it's turning from an eating disorder, finally losing the weight they have held onto, learning to love themselves and forgive events of the past, or simply becoming comfortable and confident in the body they have, there are solutions. But do you know what I have discovered? I have found that in my own life, I have to *invite* change to occur or I rebel against it. You can say you want change all you want, but talk is cheap. Change in yourself is never passive. It takes an active resolve, and can even be frightening. After all, change entails leaving behind the old you. That can be scary because you are comfortable with the "old you." That person is someone with whom you're familiar and comfortable. Saying goodbye to that person is truly like saying goodbye to a real, living person and can be very difficult, but it's also the only way to make room in your life for the person that you can become—an even better version of your already wonderful self.

What is a Healthy Lifestyle?

My idea of a healthy physical lifestyle is one that encompasses three areas:

Nutrition, Exercise, and Mental Discipline. In the following diagram, you will see my opinion on a general percentage of your efforts and how they make a difference in the way you look and feel.

This is a hierarchy of effort and application to facilitate long-lasting change in the body. Mental Discipline is the foundation on which Nutrition and Exercise are effective. Without a firm knowledge of who you are and why you deserve to treat your body with respect, focusing on the other two areas can be time spent without seeing the results you want. It's like trying to climb up a mountain of mud—you find yourself slipping and sliding all over the place without making any progress. Reaching your end goal will be very difficult if you're not properly equipped. The rope of Mental Discipline will enable you to find your grip and pull yourself up to the top of the mountain where you belong.

Truly, Mental Discipline is more important than Nutrition. Nutrition only falls into place and can be consistent enough to make permanent changes once Mental Discipline begins to sculpt your mind. The external appearance of your body is simply the reflection of the discipline in your mind. Because of observation of this relationship, I'll begin teaching you about the Power Foods Lifestyle by helping you learn about your mind, emotions, and how you view food. Only you can make change happen in your life. I can't do it for you. Neither can any doctor, trainer, or scientist— try as they might, and promise as they might. Though I can't do it for you, I will be here to teach and encourage you.

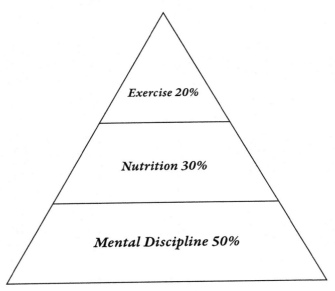

Exercise 20%

Nutrition 30%

Mental Discipline 50%

A healthy lifestyle includes caring for yourself mentally, emotionally, nutritionally, and physiologically on a daily basis. It is a combination of habits that you can maintain and continue every day for a lifetime.

What is a healthy lifestyle and how does it work in your life?

Attaining that kind of a healthy lifestyle will be a different journey for each person. There is no one-size-fits-all program. There is no miracle diet. However, there are truths. In nearly every academic study or diet approach, there are underlying principles that can be found as common threads amidst the plethora of information provided. Any principle you find that is repeated over and over again in studies may be something that can be considered truth. These are the principles I endorse, simplify, and teach in the Power Foods Lifestyle.

Will you be able to apply every principle of truth and jump right into this with 100% of your effort and resolve? Perhaps. I don't expect perfection from you, but I do expect that you will learn at least one principle from this entire book that you can use to become a better and happier person. That's all this is about—becoming a happier person.

Simplicity is the key. As you adopt and apply the principles I teach in this book, you will grow in your ability to understand your body and make wise decisions for yourself.

Strategic Routes

When you think about an airplane's flight route, it makes sense that they usually take a direct route to minimize the length of the flight. However, did you know this is only for relatively short flights? For longer inter-continental flights, the most direct route is actually not direct or a straight-line approach. Pilots follow paths that are a great circle around the curvature of the earth. If you look at a map of the world, their route will appear curved, not as a straight line from point A to point B.

Pilots take weather conditions and air currents into account in the way they approach their journey. They understand their travel will have bumps along the way and prepare for these challenges. They strategize ways to overcome any adverse weather or other conditions.

Your transition to a healthy lifestyle and healthier body is similar to these inter-continental flights. Traveling from Point A to Point B in the most direct route— like cutting as many calories as possible and spending more time exercising— may oftentimes not be the most strategic path. Obstacles will arise and you won't be able to maintain your frenzied approach. Your resolve will break, you'll "fall off the wagon," and resent yourself and your efforts. You'll wonder what's wrong with you that you can never accomplish your goal. That's because you took the straight-line approach, instead of preparing for the challenges and planning for them strategically.

Planning and preparing for these challenges doesn't prevent them from happening, but enables you to work around and through them. You will need to make adjustments and be flexible in your journey. You can learn much from "experienced pilots" who know how to best navigate from Point A to Point B. Yep, I'm comparing these pilots to my team of Body Buddies Coaches who know how to help guide you through these changes. The journey is oftentimes very long (from months to years), but you must not quit when you are over an "ocean!" You must continue with confidence toward the shore, having faith that Point B will arrive.

Face your journey with confidence, optimism, and commitment to continuing onward no matter what obstacles arise. You will experience growth, change, and the assurance that your efforts will result in reaching your final destination: a healthy body that will serve you well as you continue to care for it with a healthy lifestyle.

Your final destination may come in many forms—change of body shape, lower risk of disease, greater discipline, or increased energy. Perhaps your body does significantly change. Wonderful!

Hypothetically, how would you feel if your body did not change one inch or one pound? Would you feel your efforts were wasted? Your natural response to this question might be "Yes." Of course, you may be inclined to feel that way. But what if you were to look at it this way?

What if you knew that by changing your patterns of eating—no matter if the scale ever moved an ounce throughout the process—you were extending your life by ten years and preventing a major disease from affecting your quality of life? Would you feel your efforts were in vain then?

Remember, Body Buds, one of the most beneficial tools you can carry with you on your journey is the tool of perspective. Everything is relative. Sometimes you just need to take a step back and look at the bigger picture.

Below is a list of changes that can happen in your life as you adopt the Power Foods Lifestyle principles and seek to consistently live this way for more than 4-6 months:

- Shed excess body fat
- Overcome metabolic disorder
- Correct insulin resistance
- Manage Type 1 or Type 2 Diabetes
- Reduce cholesterol
- Strengthen functions of vital organs
- Reduce risk of heart disease
- Reduce risk of pre-diabetes
- Experience greater energy levels
- Reduce emotional dependence on food
- Cope with daily stress more effectively
- Reduce symptoms of anxiety and depression
- Increase self-respect and self-confidence
- Gain a more positive perspective

How Long Will It Take?

The trick to starting this lifestyle change is to dedicate two months (eight weeks) to this lifestyle, being sure to follow every recommendation as closely as possible. This is the only way you will truly reap the benefits of how the PFL trains your body and your mind. After your initial eight weeks of dedicated learning (think of it as your training course), you will have learned enough to continue eating how you feel is best for your body and maintaining the implementation of principles that work for you. You should feel independent from numbers and counting, feeling confident in the way you view food, and can strategically eat as a way of life.

If you decide to return to your old habits of eating, you will probably feel a stark difference in your body. You will feel less energy, less control, and less vitality. You will realize just how much higher quality of life you enjoy when you are eating nutrients in proper balance to provide your body with energy, staying physically active, and exercising control over your mind. At the end of training yourself on the PFL, you will feel a great enthusiasm about your body and the discipline you have attained. You will notice the changes in your body, mindset, and energy flow. I hope you will decide that this lifestyle is one you wish to continue. Regardless of whether you are working toward your goal or not, time will pass. Will you have improvements physically and mentally to show for that time?

Adopting a healthy lifestyle can be done by taking baby steps. These baby steps are small changes that you can maintain over a long period of time and lead to great results. This journey is worth making. I applaud you for your desire to give this your best effort. Please don't expect perfection of yourself. Take those baby steps forward, make small and maintainable changes, and be sure to acknowledge your progress. Any movement forward is movement in the right direction.

You do not need to be following the structure 100% in order to be living a Power Foods Lifestyle. You are living the PFL when you seek to combine foods strategically, when you keep your portions smaller, when you drink lots of water, when you exercise, and when you cook more at home than you dine out. Don't be afraid of failure. There are many levels at which you can live the principles I teach in this book. Choose your level and intensity and go for it! I've designed this to be empowering and increase your awareness, not a method designed for you to feel like a failure because you can't live it to the tee. The guidelines I give are the ideal—not the expectation.

I wrote this entire book for you—to help you reach a frame of mind wherein you believe that you can do this. You can change your life. You can be in control. You can love healthy foods. You can make good choices. You can form new habits. You can be the master of your thoughts and behaviors. Knowledge is power, but knowledge in action is unstoppable.

The first two weeks of living the PFL will take extra work and investment of your time. It's important that you plan and prepare to change your daily habits in order to accommodate your new lifestyle. After these initial weeks, however, you will have developed a routine and a pattern of success. From that point on, much less thought will be needed because you have already formed appropriate habits. It does get easier!

You can't fail unless you give up and stop trying. The intensity of living the PFL you pursue should be maintainable and sustainable. Some days will be easier than others. No matter whether it's easy or hard, I will be here for you cheering you on. Throughout the remainder of this book, I will provide many tips and strategies for you to consider as you make your lifestyle change. I want you to make this work for you.

I can't promise you that adopting a PFL lifestyle will be the easiest thing you have done, but I can promise you that you will develop discipline and control that impacts every part of your life. You will be so proud of yourself. You will push through barriers and obstacles you never knew you had the strength to overcome. You will be ready to make principles of the PFL a part of your life for the rest of your life.

This is not a diet.
This is not a quick-fix.
This is not for a short span of time.
This is about change.
This is about health.
This is about knowledge.
This is about your ability to make your own choices.
This is about consistency.
This is about maintaining and sustaining good choices.
These are true principles, proven over and
over and over again.
This is a lifestyle.
This is the Power Foods Lifestyle.

Time to get to work.

2
Mental Discipline

How many doctors are overweight?
How many financial advisors are in debt?
How many beauticians have damaged hair?

There can be professionals everywhere who lack the ability to follow and apply everything they know on an intellectual level. I don't say this to tear individuals down—I say this to show that any of us can have all the knowledge in the world, yet not use it for our benefit. Until we apply it to mold our behavior, that knowledge will only take us so far.

In this chapter I will address many of the emotional and mental obstacles we each face on a daily basis and suggest ideas of how we might overcome them. As an individual who struggled for years with disordered eating and the resulting self-loathing for being unable to break the cycle, I've had to consistently put forth effort to temper my own emotional and mental obstacles. I am so pleased with my progress that has taken place in the past three years, and owe much of it to the growth of Body Buddies and so many of you—the amazing people with whom I'm blessed to share my story. Knowing each member of the Body Buddies family out there is fighting for improvement has kept me going through the tough times that I have doubted myself. Thank you for joining this family—we are all in the trenches together!

No matter how long you have allowed negativity to be a part of your life, you can overcome the mental blocks that are most prevalent. It will take consistent effort and awareness to change the patterns of your thoughts, but it's very possible. You are more than capable once you realize only your thoughts and beliefs define you.

I hope you'll do more than just read this chapter. I hope you'll pause often to reflect on your life and the obstacles that hold you back. This information will only be effective as you take time for thorough self-analysis. If introspection is a new concept for you, digging inside your emotions and thoughts may feel a little awkward at first. It's not every day that you try to dissect your emotions to analyze what's actually going on in there. Most people prefer to stuff them away and pretend they don't exist. The problem with this, however, is that lack of resolution can later impact your subconscious mind—the underlying thought patterns that dominate the conscious mind. This is how you can talk and talk and talk about making a change, yet then go pig out on a pizza and brownies! This explains a lot, doesn't it? So let's open up your mind and start paying attention to what's going on, and seek to re-program any thought patterns that will be better off where that pizza and brownies belong—in the garbage. (Unless it's an indulgence meal, of course. . . read on to learn more.)

Rest assured that you will quickly improve at introspection as you practice. Let's test out a hypothetical situation (that may actually be factual for you) to get the hang of tracing your emotions and thoughts:

*　　　*　　　*　　　*　　　*

It's a Tuesday morning and you're running late. You open your closet, pick out an article of clothing you think might work for the day, and then try it on. After analyzing your image in the mirror, you furiously strip the clothing off your body while mentally growling: fat, fat, and fat. You then try another article of clothing and the same thing happens. A look of disgust clouds your face. This time, the voice is meaner. *You are so fat and gross. How could you let this happen?*

*　　　*　　　*　　　*　　　*

I hope you're laughing with me as surely you and I both have had our fair share of those days! I'm sure you'll agree that there is nothing more disruptive to what may have been a productive and positive day than for these negative voices to beat you down. Your feelings of disgust and frustration often spill over into the remainder of your day's activities and you become pessimistic, snippy, and lack an overall excitement for life. Attitudes really are contagious, and this is an attitude that's not worth catching.

In this situation, you might arrive at the end of your day, eating foods to cope with your negative emotions, and wonder why you had such an awful day. Well, let's back track from the behavior through the emotion and the thoughts.

Behavior: Eating non-strategic foods that make you feel poorly about yourself and don't improve your health. Moodiness and pessimistic attitude toward others.

Now let's trace what initiated that behavior.

Emotion: Feeling anger and resentment toward yourself for poor health choices over the months and years. Disappointment. Sadness. Anger.

These emotions are what triggered the behavior, the need to do something to cope with these uncomfortable feelings instead of acknowledging them with an open heart and mind. So where did the emotion come from? Emotions don't just magically appear.

Thought: The thoughts that you allowed in your mind from that morning when trying on clothes: "I'm so fat." "I'm unattractive." "I feel and look gross."

It doesn't make you a weak person to have these negative thoughts. However, it is critical that you re-frame those thoughts and shift them into positive thoughts.

By refusing to do so, you invite the resulting negative emotion to be a part of your life, which then influences your behavior. This cycle will be perpetuated for your entire life until you make the decision to change your thoughts the instant negativity enshrouds your mind.

This three-step process of back-tracking from your behavior to the initial trigger thought(s) can help you improve other elements of your life as well. I hope you're learning a lot and taking time to stop and think about what thoughts tend to be a part of your life. Perhaps some of these other voices plague you as well:

- *I'm already fat so why should I even try?*
- *Everyone already expects me to eat garbage, so I should.*
- *If people see me eating healthily, they will wonder why I am so big.*
- *I'm already miserable so I may as well eat something delicious and enjoy my misery. Why be fat and unhappy?*
- *There's no point to changing my habits—I don't have the willpower to change for good.*

- *What's wrong with me? Nothing motivates me to try harder. I just don't have the motivation or desire.*

All of these thoughts can begin a landslide of negative emotions. Together, these "downer" thoughts lead to the behaviors that ostracize you from landmarks of progress. Most of the time, it's by turning to comfort food or a full-out binge that will not only halt your progress in caring for your health, but take you a step backward in your conscious confidence to make wise decisions.

You can succeed in training your mind to think differently. You can succeed in changing your behavior. It all starts with recognition. Use this next section to help you learn to recognize the triggers that are most impacting you.

Identifying Emotional Triggers

Life is an invitation for you to experience roller coasters of emotions. You can be up high, down low, swinging far left, and curving right. You can be all over the place!

This doesn't make the emotions the problem; the problem is that you all too readily deal with your emotional issues using food, which is why diets have such a high rate of failure. Over the course of your life, you will experience that roller coaster of emotions frequently. Emotions hijack you of your resolve and determination to succeed with the tools and knowledge you have about nutrition and exercise. So if your emotions are all over the place, does that mean your eating patterns and physical health are doomed?

Emotional eating has occurred in your life if you have ever made room for dessert although you're already full, or gone searching for chocolate or those potato chips when you're feeling down. When you use food to make you feel better and fill your emotional needs instead of your stomach's needs, you set yourself up for negative associations with food. Your health and confidence in yourself may then plummet as, deep down, you know you aren't handling your emotions in appropriate ways. You may consciously or only subconsciously experience this. Eating will never fix the way you feel; instead, it will simply exacerbate the feelings of negativity you are experiencing.

Now I need to clarify something—I'm not saying that food is bad! Goodness gracious, we all love food! Using food occasionally as a reward or celebration is an awesome thing. However, food can become a hole in the boat of your life when eating is your primary emotional coping mechanism—when your first impulse is to open the refrigerator or stop by your favorite fast food restaurant whenever you're upset, angry, lonely, stressed, exhausted, or bored. You will wind up trapped in an unhealthy cycle where the real feeling or problem is never addressed. How can you fix the problem if you refuse to acknowledge it?

As you seek to improve your health using the strategies of the Power Foods Lifestyle, you will most likely be sabotaged by something sooner or later. It's quite often that a client, while being coached through their lifestyle change, will experience a major life event. I am so pleased with those who didn't give up and say, 'I can't take this.' Instead, these clients used their new eating and exercise behaviors to create a new coping mechanism. Acknowledging that obstacles exist and will, most likely, find you sooner or later should help you to strategize ways to maneuver safely around them while still striving for your goals.

Gaining greater awareness of your emotional and mental state is a daily task, and one that should continue moving up on your priority list. Practice doesn't make perfect, but it does invite progress. With control and discipline over your mind, you can give yourself the freedom to be happy, confident, and to achieve all of your goals.

Discouraging People

Getting together with other people for a meal is a great way to relieve stress and build relationships, but it can also lead to social overeating. Overindulging can happen simply because the food is there and you're sitting at the table for a longer period of time, because everyone else is eating, or because you have deprived yourself too drastically with weight loss efforts and end up losing your willpower. I think those are some of the most frustrating times as you want to eat the delicious and very satisfying, yet non-strategic foods, but you're angry at yourself as you know you have just derailed your progress. "I had a big setback," is the way that clients have often described that situation to me.

You may also overeat in social situations out of nervousness or shyness—to keep yourself busy so you don't have to talk to anyone. Perhaps your family or circle of friends encourages you to overeat with their own habits and traditions, and it's easier to go along with the group than to cause a rift by your non-compliance.

The majority of those around you will probably applaud your efforts and seek to help you as you begin your healthy lifestyle. However, be aware that even those closest to you may unintentionally attract you away from your goals. As they see your efforts to improve your life, a very bright spotlight may shine on their own insecurities and lack of discipline in their own life. Due to their feelings of guilt and displeasure with themselves, they might subconsciously attempt to bring you down through their discouraging or taunting words.

But you're already thin!
C'mon now, stop making the rest of us feel bad by eating like that.

One meal won't hurt! Just this once...
I made it just for you because I know it's your favorite!

In most cases, their intentions are not to purposely tear you down or sabotage you. Forgive them for their lack of awareness, though your initial urge might be to retaliate and get defensive, or be weak and give in. I have seen many people bend in their commitment and give in to their old lifestyle habits because they couldn't handle the negative opposition. Seek not to be one of these people. Stand firm in your resolution to make a change for you in your life. Decide to be stronger more often.

There is a saying in the fitness world that many athletes and very dedicated people use: "haters gonna hate." I think this is a horribly-coined phrase, though the meaning behind it resonates. Yes, there will be people who might not be happy and giddy about your success as you change your body, but don't seek to fight them. This will only contaminate your relationship with them and drive a wedge into your commitment to your new lifestyle.

Perhaps avoiding these types of people is not an option—this person may be your spouse or someone else very close to you. So then what do you do? I'd like to tell you a story and let you create your own conclusion for your personal situation:

When initially working to transform my body in the spring of 2012, I was following an extremely difficult meal plan. The fat was melting off my body so quickly that my family and friends were all raising their eyebrows. For the most part, no one except my roommates and co-workers saw what I ate (which was not too exciting—trust me). But when I visited my family in my hometown and was turning down even "healthy" food like roast beef, baked potatoes, beets, and corn in place of chicken, green vegetables, and avocado, I began to hear some concerned comments. My family didn't understand why I was turning down "healthy" food. It seemed I had become a food snob and this attitude was creating a disturbance in the normal and comfortable routine of family mealtime. I endured three more weeks of comments and slight allegations of obsessiveness that then began coming from my friends and co-workers as well.

"Don't you ever get to eat anything fun? I'm so glad I'm not you."
"You're no fun anymore. We can't even go out to eat with you..."
"Want a piece of this? Oh wait . . . you can't have this. Ha ha!"
"You're taking this overboard. You're starting to worry me. . ."

These types of phrases were very hurtful in the beginning. I knew why I was doing what I was doing, yet no one seemed to be happy that I was conquering my weak-willed self and getting closer and closer to my end goal. No one was rejoicing in my successes with me. Shouldn't they have been happy for me? Didn't they know how much progress I was making? Weren't they aware that I was finally mastering my negative cycles of binge eating and feeling angry with myself? The fact is, they didn't know. I hadn't communicated with them the true purpose for my goal, nor why I had taken it to the level of discipline I had.

To make matters worse, this all happened at the same time my oldest brother took his life, which was a very traumatic event for my family and me. Many of the people who love me considered my new focus and habits to be my way of coping with the pain and feelings of sadness and loss. But they weren't. In fact, Denzel's death helped me continue in my resolve to correct my life. I knew that he would have wanted me to conquer myself. I knew he would be proud of me. My efforts made me feel that I was actually closer to him than before. He was, after all, the first person who taught me how to lift weights correctly. I had even spent time with him at his home two weeks prior to his death and told him my "secret," that I was going to compete in a Women's Figure competition. He had encouraged me to continue striving for my goal, and reminded me that it didn't matter what anyone thought except for myself. I will always remember him telling me to be my idea of my best self, and stop trying to please everyone else. I remembered this, and harnessed those thoughts in my mind.

My family and friends didn't know Denzel's exit from our lives was actually a motivating factor until six weeks into my body transformation. At that time, I finally sat down with my mom on the steps outside the front door of my parents' home.

"Mom," I confided, "can I tell you why I'm doing what I'm doing?" She nodded, and listened quietly.

"Did you know that from the time I was nine years old, I've been concerned about my weight and the way I looked? Did you know that I have loathed myself for years because I didn't have the body that I knew I was capable of achieving? Did you know that all those years in front of the mirror in the dance studio made me feel I was never good enough? Were you aware that I have struggled with disordered eating and exercise, and tried to conquer my demons, for the past fourteen years? Did you know that I have felt like the biggest failure for too long?"

The external actions of my sixteen-year trial were evident to nearly everyone who knew me—I was constantly going to the gym, constantly on a diet, and constantly talking about losing weight. Everyone just thought I was a health nut! But a thorough explanation of my long-held deeper issues—binge-eating, yo-yo dieting, and excessive/obsessive exercise—were what helped my mom to understand what had happened internally during that time.

"Kristy, I had no idea you were dealing with any of this," she said. "Why couldn't you have just told me?" Of course, my mom was very much aware of my desires to be fit, healthy, and trim, but the inner struggles were the non-communicated point.

I learned an important lesson that day. I learned that it is very important to share your reasons for putting so much effort into changing your behaviors with those closest to you. They love you. They will try to understand. They can't read your mind and automatically understand your deepest feelings and motivation. Discussing your reasons for change, fears, goals, and small triumphs with those you love might be the key to not only eliminating effort-sabotaging comments, but building a support system around you.

If you choose to do this, remember that the outcome may not always be like my story where a mutual understanding was achieved. In the event that the person with whom you are sharing your innermost thoughts doesn't understand and still elicits your anger and defensiveness, you must remember why you're working to change your eating behavior. This is for you and your health. It's also for those you love—even if they don't see it as that. You are extending your life and greatly enhancing the quality of that life through every meal in which you focus on putting good nutrients in your body. You are giving yourself confidence—not only physically in the way you look, but through your discipline and choices. You are giving yourself permission to be a happier person (biochemically speaking, this is true! Your moods will be far better than if your eating lacks structure and strategy) which will influence the happiness of the people around you. Your purpose is a great one.

Being Too Busy

The statement of "I'm just too busy" is arguably the top excuse I hear from people who aren't quite ready to give their health the attention it deserves. "Busily" is the way you probably live your life.

- Too busy to cook
- Too busy to grocery shop
- Too busy to plan
- Too busy to exercise
- Too busy for anything

Do you know the one thing in life that is fair?
We each have 24 hours in a day.

The way you spend your time each day determines who and what you become. Here's a deep question I would like you to consider for a few moments: Do you love what you are currently doing with your 24 hours so much that you don't mind only doing it until your body shuts down? The current statistics for health and risk of disease aren't looking too bright for those who don't take control, so it all comes down to priorities. How can you continue living your busy life if you don't have the health to do it? What are you worth then? Health comes void of a price tag. It's time to beat the trend of waiting until there is a problem or dire necessity to make a change.

Stress

Have you ever noticed how stress makes you hungry? Oddly enough, I find that I have the hardest time controlling my appetite when I have the most going on. It's like my mind kicks into overdrive and I feel like I should be eating at every possible second to calm my nerves. It's during these times that handfuls of M&Ms, potato chips, French fries, cookies, and anything else with sugar and fat passes my mouth without me even batting any eye or realizing what I'm doing. Can you relate to this?

When stress is chronic as it so often is in our chaotic, fast-paced world, high levels of the stress hormone, Cortisol, are produced. Cortisol triggers cravings for salty, sweet, and high-fat foods because they give you a burst of energy and pleasure. The more you have uncontrolled stress in your life, the more likely you are to turn to non-strategic foods for emotional relief.

I believe that one of the best ways to combat unnecessary eating is by planning your meals. This doesn't take more than 5-10 minutes each night, or longer for the week ahead on Sunday. As you learn the details of and follow the PFL, you will have approximately six pre-planned meals per day. As you become structured and methodical in the fueling of your body, any desires to eat outside of your allotted meals and food times can easily be recognized as an emotionally-triggered event (fixation), not an event triggered by hunger or nutritional necessity (craving). When you realize that you're experiencing an emotionally-triggered fixation, you can begin the process of working through the feelings logically, instead of masking them by putting food to your mouth.

Relationship Woes

They can be the best and the worst thing in the entire world. Feelings of loss that occur when you lose somebody close to you through divorce, death, break-up, or infidelity cannot be understood entirely by any other person. Your grief and pain is individual. You are built to interact with others and to share bonds that are woven with emotions. When these bonds are broken, you feel robbed, cheated, and angry. You feel hurt.

These emotions are real. Never feel ashamed of your emotions. It's okay to feel deeply. It's okay to cry. Your tears are evidence of just how deeply you love. Loving is a noble characteristic and one you must never be afraid to give again, even when it can seem beyond your capabilities.

Where do you turn when these very difficult emotions surface? It's pretty common understanding that the "cure" for many women's emotional woes is chocolate, where men's cure is a steak, or even a bowl of ice cream. Perhaps it's a bottle of wine or other variety of alcohol. We all have our comfort foods or beverages that give us a temporary high and a feeling of pleasure. For just a few moments, your mind is relieved of the burdensome emotions that constantly torment you. It's your way of escaping. But sadly, the guilt and feelings of sickness or disappointment soon follow, and then you feel a double negative emotion—first the relationship feelings, then the feelings of disgust and physical discomfort from what you just put in your body.

To make matters worse, choosing to follow a healthy lifestyle may feel like you have lost yet another endearing relationship. You have a special and unique relationship with food. It brings you happiness and feelings of familiarity and comfort. So when you feel that's taken away—like your relationship—it's very easy to feel angry and even resentful. You subconsciously will strive to get one of those relationships back, and that is food. After all, at least you can control whether food is in your life or not, unlike relationships with people.

One of the best remedies for this situation is to think through a few strategic "treats" that are not going to disrupt your efforts in your healthy lifestyle, yet help you still feel like you are allowing yourself that splurge. There is something healing in allowing yourself comfort in the form of food, but it doesn't need to be something that undermines your health.

For example, my all-time favorite comfort food has always been peanut butter and honey/jelly sandwiches. When I was young, I became fearful a lot during the nights—of the dark . . . of ghosts . . . of monsters . . . I was a frightened child. So what did I use to comfort myself? I quietly tip-toed from my basement bedroom up the stairs to the pantry, closed the door, turned on the light, and made a triple-decker PB sandwich using soft, white, fluffy bread. After my sandwich was prepared, I then turned off the light before opening the pantry door, tip-toed down the stairs, then indulged in my favorite food in the comfort of my bed. It made me feel safe, secure, and happy. I did this probably once a week for many years.

This relationship has been my go-to my whole life, including when I first arrived in Seoul, Korea as a new missionary for the Church of Jesus Christ of Latter-day Saints (the "Mormons"). I couldn't eat Korean food for the life of me! Just the smell of kimchi—which seemed to permeate the very air around me—made me sick to my stomach. Thankfully, I was given normal bread and peanut butter from caring friends who had access to the military base. Once again, my relationship with PB&J made me feel safe, secure, and comforted in such an unfamiliar and difficult situation and environment.

Peanut butter sandwiches are not inherently bad, but the reasons I turned to them were not for nutrition, but as a coping mechanism. Additionally, what I didn't know then is that the combination of carbohydrates + fats + sugar (oh my, the power poison! You'll learn more as you continue reading this book) wouldn't help me improve the shape of my body and feel good about myself. I have had to re-train my mind over the last few years to associate a new food as my go-to for comfort. So what has replaced peanut butter sandwiches?

A peanut butter protein shake that soothes me, yet doesn't bring me guilt:

- 2 cups warm water
- 2 scoops chocolate protein powder
- 1 Tbsp. 100% natural Peanut Butter
- 1 tsp. Honey

What are your comfort foods? One of the most helpful ways to spend five minutes of your time is to brainstorm a list of better options that you can eat when your willpower is down due to emotions. I often have had clients post a small list on the side of the fridge to use when they experience these feelings. Can you brainstorm ways to satisfy and comfort yourself without damaging your healthy lifestyle? It's very possible, just requires some creativity and forethought. Be sure to include some of the sweet treat ideas from the Power Foods Lifestyle Recipe Books.

Depression and Sadness

You may occasionally experience events that bring you sadness and even put you in a state of depression. It's normal to want to cope with those emotions by hiding and ignoring them. But it's not okay to turn to foods that impair your health and your view of yourself as a person. Eating unhealthy foods in large quantities is not the problem—it is the symptom. The problem is not knowing how to cope with the feelings you have.

When you feel down and sad, you have two choices. You can either let the negative emotions win, or you can choose to focus on the things that are going well in your life. Take some time to sit and make a list of all the blessings, conveniences, and happiness in your life. They may be as monumental as marrying the person you love, or something as trivial as the cat finally remembering to use its litter box. What has gone right? What has surprised you? What has made you smile? What have others done for you lately? You might be surprised at how many items appear on your list when you think about it for more than a few moments.

During the years I was growing up, my mom kept a large notebook on the kitchen counter of our home. Each morning, my six siblings and I wrote down one thing for which we were grateful. Now years later, we look back over those notebooks and laugh about the things we recorded. While sometimes silly items appeared like socks, milk, no homework, toys, no oatmeal for breakfast, or "only had to practice the piano for half an hour," they were items that we could have easily overlooked if we hadn't been given the opportunity to think about them.

I challenge you to keep a gratitude notebook and record a few things each day that make you realize how blessed and fortunate you are. As one of the laws of the universe states, by showing gratitude, you demonstrate that you can attract more positivity to your life.

Slow Results

The PFL's strategic approach to changing your body from the inside out may feel quite blasé—almost like you're not doing enough. To some, it even feels counter-intuitive to what society has trained you to believe about weight loss and dieting. This is true especially if you're prone to fad diets and taking society's extreme measures. Those types of efforts alone are one of the greatest reasons people have become frustrated and given up before—they don't see the results they desire, even when pushing hard.

The science of how the body sheds fat is quite complicated and involves many variables. However, let's keep it simple for now:

To lose weight, you must create a caloric deficit. This means you need to put less into your body than you expend in energy (calories). In those terms, we associate a deficit of 3,500 calories with one pound of body weight. The problem, though, lies in hormones, metabolism, genetics, and thyroid health. Due to these factors, there is no specific answer to why your weight can fluctuate the way it does. Add into all of this the fact that the glycogen and water storage in our bodies can fluctuate 5–10 pounds based on the food and water consumed and the time of day. This means that eating a heavy dinner and drinking a lot of water the night before weighing can make you think you gained weight, though you did not.

Measurements may or may not change due to change in body composition.

I see it all the time—clients who have a phenomenal change in the look and shape of their physique, but never lose a pound or change more than a few quarters of an inch in measurements. What do I mean when I say body composition? I'm talking about the ratio of lean muscle tissue to body fat. The better composition someone has, the more muscle they will have in proportion to the amount of fat. I don't put any stock in body fat measurements. I haven't had a body fat test in over three years and am not interested in having one performed as studies show they can vary greatly. Why would I put that stimulus in my mind to either "incentivize" myself to continue making changes, or use fear and disparage over a silly number? No. I worked too long and hard to clear my mind of that focus.

Instead, I choose to use these tools to measure how I'm doing:
- Photo progress
- The fit of my clothes
- My level of adherence and discipline

I truly wish to see you do this as well, but know that it takes time to reach that level of emotional separation. Numbers on the scale are used simply as '*oh, that's interesting moments,*' but never as a means to be happy or sad. I choose to keep my emotions 100% independent from numbers and use the three bullet points above to gauge progress. Again, it takes time to develop this separation and freedom, but is possible if you truly wish to attain it.

You can start generating this freedom from results, and begin focusing on progress and effort through the following steps:

1. Get rid of the scale—just don't use it. Many of my clients are not allowed to weigh when I learn how obsessive their behavior is. I explain how important it is for them to focus on behavioral changes, and so we never know their weight throughout their entire program, which can be anywhere from 8 to 48 weeks.

2. Measure your body every two to four weeks at the same time of day.
   a. Chest
   b. Waist
   c. Hips (fullest part)
   d. Inner thigh (right side)
   e. Quad (right side, 4" up from the top of the knee)
   f. Calves (right side, foot flat on ground at fullest part)
   g. Bicep (right side, arm extended and palm up with a relaxed muscle)

3. Stop doing body fat tests (unless this truly is the only thing that will motivate you to make a change.) I hope to see you transition to being motivated through the desire to care for your body.

4.Take bi-weekly or monthly progress photos. Wear the same clothing at the same time of day with the same lighting. Stand with your arms to your sides with good posture. Hold yourself upright, but do not flex. Smile, as you are working to change your body. Take a photo of the front, back, and side views of your body. Keep your photos in a file to compare. Having a recurring "photo day" in your calendar or tasking system is helpful to keep you on track.

As you begin focusing on the behavior, the results will come—but with time. I'm going to be very blunt with you: the Power Foods Lifestyle is not a quick-fix. You will not drop five pounds in one week. If that's what you are looking for, you will be severely disappointed. I wish to always be the pragmatic voice in an industry of deceptive manipulation, and will do my best to help you steer clear from the ruse of this industry's marketing as I further educate you.

Although the PFL won't cause "miraculous results" in 10 days, it will produce "miraculous results" in the long run. You will train your mind and your body to expect nutrients in balance. It will help reduce fat mass on your body to an amount that is healthy and maintainable. It will create a new level of energy, personal control, and satisfaction that will lead to the fit and healthy body you've dreamed of.

Many of my clients who begin this lifestyle approach me in the first two weeks with sullen expressions and frustration as they are not dropping weight as quickly as they thought. I console them, explaining that their body is changing one cell at a time, and that true physical change takes time. Consistency in this lifestyle is king! The body will change, but it takes time as it figures out the process. Consider how long you have trained your body to react as it currently is. It didn't happen overnight, did it? Might I suggest it is even disrespectful to your body that works so hard in your behalf to change so quickly the instant you change the variables? Perhaps you should remember your body is intelligent, and will evolve to meet the needs of the consistent variables you place upon it. This will help you generate more patience in making the change—and keeping it.

When I explain this to clients of the Body Buddies Coaching system, they usually return to their efforts and follow the principles of the lifestyle, determined to continue being consistent. Fast forward to one month, then two months, then six months down the road, and these people achieve the bodies and health status they have dreamed of in the most healthy and strategic way possible. They truly change their bodies from the inside out, at a pace slow enough to develop habits and consistency for life-long maintenance. They correct metabolic damage and insulin resistance. They have more energy and they 'wow' their doctors when they have their next annual wellness exam. They learn to recognize food as fuel. They know how to plan their meals and take responsibility for themselves. They no longer rely on me or a product (we ex-nay the use of shakes, wraps, pills, or other products that don't fit the principles of the PFL.) Their character and habits are now a product of their efforts. They truly have adapted to the Power Foods Lifestyle.

Whether you are coached through the process or are able to apply it on your own with the help of this book and all of the other resources I give, I hope you will experience everything I mentioned above. I want that for you so badly, but I know my wanting it for you isn't enough. You have to put forth the effort and keep yourself focused on the long-term picture. For that reason, I encourage you to return to this book often, perhaps dog-earing and highlighting sections you feel will be good for you to re-visit. You are capable. You have it inside of you. Your doubts and fears can be dispelled as you focus on baby steps. You are already on your way!

Conclusion

As you gain consistency at putting health-supporting nutrients in your body, you will be greatly enhancing your quality of life. Remember to focus on behavior, not results. You are doing all in your power to change the way you look, feel, and behave. View your self-sabotage and self-anger as the next challenge to overcome. How can you do it?

• Try placing sticky notes around your house. On those notes, write about how proud of your efforts you are. Acknowledge your amazing attributes. Flaunt your positive qualities. This can become a very fun and confidence-boosting activity.

• I have an ever-present note on my fridge that reads: "Your journey is your journey, and your journey alone." Constantly seeing reminders like this helps me to remain focused and centered on my goals. I know this can help you, too. Seeing the positive aspects of who you are trying to become will help transform the fabric of your mind.

• Try memorizing quotes you can repeat out loud to yourself when you start to feel down about your efforts. Here are several of my favorites I have memorized:

"If you always put limits on everything you do, physical or anything else, it will spread into your work and into your life. There are no limits. There are only plateaus, and you must not stay there, you must go beyond them."
—*Bruce Lee*

"Twenty years from now you will be more disappointed by the things that you didn't do than by the ones you did do, so throw off the bowlines, sail away from safe harbor, catch the trade winds in your sails. Explore. Dream. Discover."
—*Mark Twain*

"I am not a product of my circumstances. I am a product of my decisions."
—*Stephen Covey*

Many of the people with whom I have worked experience the great relief that comes through journaling and identifying their emotions daily. If you have never been one to write your thoughts and feelings down on paper, it can initially be a very daunting task. Digging inside your thoughts for what you are truly thinking and feeling can be scary. But I'd like you to try to do it.

Start with writing one sentence. You need to reveal who you truly are, and only when you see it in writing can you better analyze the tone of voice you allow inside your mind. By beginning to journal your emotions as a part of your new lifestyle, you will experience a new power you never knew you had.

To begin journaling, try writing down several sentences that answer the following questions:

1. What foods sound very appealing to you at this moment? Why do you think that is?
2. What is the biggest stress on your mind?
3. Who are you worried about?
4. What is making you afraid?
5. What has happened recently that makes you sad?
6. What is occupying your time and keeping you from caring for your health?

Look over the sentences you wrote and see if you can identify any of the emotional triggers we have talked about in this chapter. Can you use the resources to face these thoughts and feelings? I know you can. You are a strong person. You are becoming better every single day.

It will take practice to develop this "muscle" of control in your mind. It may be years that you have stuffed your emotions deep within, refusing to look at what's happening inside of you. As you utilize the tools and strategies in this chapter, I hope you can begin conquering these habits one by one. Columbus didn't cross the ocean in a day! Keep that in mind as you forge ahead in making progress in your own life. No matter how young or not-so-young you are, you can re-train your mind. You can change your habits.

Be very careful not to expect perfection of yourself. Remember, this is a lifestyle change, not something that happens in a day or a few weeks! You may find that you take a few steps forward, but then a couple of steps backward. As long as you continue trying, that is all that matters!

Commend yourself for being brave and willing to face your inner opposition. It's a hard thing to actually voice the problem, but there is much power in it as well. Until you are ready to face your challenges head-on, change can't occur in your life. It's time to plow ahead. You are ready to take yourself on—to set goals, to discipline your mind, and to form new and life-changing habits. This is your chance to improve your mind and body for life.

Focus on behavior, not results.

3
Setting Goals

Efforts to change your body can feel like a total waste of time when you don't see immediate results. This is why it's extremely important to become really good at setting goals—and small, attainable ones!

One of the most prevalent forms of self-sabotage I see in people working to change their bodies and health involves setting a number of pounds to lose. For example, saying, "I will lose 20 pounds by April 1st." The problem with this is not in setting the goal. Nor is it in putting a stamp of time on the goal. The problem lies in the fact that weight loss (and let's correct that—fat loss) is not a straight-line event. And if the goal doesn't happen, especially at the speed you wish to see it happen, you might find yourself giving up on the approach and returning to your former way of life.

Sounds pretty familiar, right? That's because this is how most people have programmed themselves to think and react. Surely you are no exception. So let's tweak the thoughts and reactions.

Focus on Consistent Behavior, and the Results Will Come

Instead of focusing on a number of pounds to lose—which is simply a result of new behaviors—learn to focus your mind on the behavior that needs to change. You will only get results when you change your actions and keep them consistent. Your body wants to function optimally, but it can only do that with a certain combination of variables that are consistently placed upon it. Your body is quite an intelligent creation. Throughout the remainder of this book, you will learn strategies that will help your body use that intelligence to improve your health. Does that mean you'll be perfect at them? No. But the key here is to get really good at picking yourself up and trying again. That is the consistency you need to foster if you want long-term change—a true lifestyle change.

You may have formerly become angry with yourself with a stubborn number on the scale. We all have! I really think if each of us threw a scale out the window every time we wanted to, there would be no scales in any homes on this earth!

I'd like to present a new thought to you: have you ever thought about how disrespectful to yourself it is to be angry at lack of change if you're not focusing on consistently making that change? You see, you can't eat a certain healthful way for 5-10 days and expect this incredible change. Your body has just started to realize that, hey, there is a change in the variables it's getting. It might need to think about adjusting the way it functions—perhaps synthesizing some new lean muscle tissue, utilizing stored adipose tissue for fat, etc. Be kind to your body! It's done the best it can with the variables you have consistently given it.

Have you been a yo-yo dieter? Well then, yeah, your body is a bit confused. Have you often deprived yourself of food? Then yeah, your body is going to be more apt to store food when you feed yourself. Your body will respond over time, but you must learn to be consistent. You will become consistent when you get very good at setting small goals—working to change your behavior, rather than hyper-focusing on results.

Where to Begin

Successful people think about their goals constantly. They write them down, set up a reminder for themselves, and get the obstacles out of the way so they can achieve those goals. Only a small number of people actually write their goals down. An even smaller number of people actually place their goals where they can see them every day. I hope you commit to becoming one of the minority.

Goal setting is the means by which you can accomplish your dreams that otherwise would remain unrealized. I'm sure you've heard the phrase:

Fail to plan, plan to fail.

It's true! How can you expect yourself to realize progress if you don't know what you are striving to accomplish? How can you remain committed to your program without a way to measure your progress? It's time to put an end to your lack of goal setting, and make this characteristic your new strength.

Your experience with setting goals may be astronomical or absolutely minimal. It doesn't matter. I'd like to show you what I find to be the best strategy for keeping yourself balanced in life while still progressing toward your goals. I'll walk you through the process of how to set your goals each week, then each month.

Weekly Goal Setting

Spend 5-10 minutes setting your goals and writing them down. I encourage my clients to set an alarm on their phone or calendar to go off on Sunday evenings, reminding them to set their goals. I ask them to make a small, simple goal for each of the four areas:

1. Nutrition
2. Fitness
3. Mindset
4. Spiritual

After working with so many individuals, I have truly found that these four areas of goals work synergistically to produce so much happiness—no matter a person's background. Here's an example of what I might see a client write down and hang on their computer monitor, save as their phone's lock screen, or write on a 3x5 card to place on the dashboard of their car:

1. I will be cautious about carbs at night and seek to replace them with Power Fats.
2. I will be diligent in my scheduled cardio sessions and give them 100% effort.
3. I will be aware of negative thoughts and seek to re-frame them into positive thoughts.
4. I will spend 10 minutes daily in spiritual study or meditation.

The most important part of your weekly goals is that they are bite-size chunks of your monthly goals, which I will share next. Your week will be productive and beneficial as you focus on these four, doable tasks. Setting new goals should also reflect a desire to overcome the greatest obstacle you faced in the previous week.

"You don't set out to build a wall. You don't say 'I'm going to build the biggest, baddest, greatest wall that's ever been built.' You don't start there. You say, 'I'm going to lay this brick as perfectly as a brick can be laid.' You do that every single day. And soon you have a wall."
—*Will Smith*

Monthly Goal Setting

Spend 15-20 minutes doing this exercise and begin stepping confidently toward your goals! The time you spend setting goals is a direct investment in yourself. Make time to sit quietly and plan. For every step in this process, take a moment to write down your thoughts. This will be very important for you to look back on later.

1. Take a clean sheet of paper.

2. Think about one goal you would like to accomplish.
   - Example: Lose 10 lbs.

This should be the maximum amount of weight to lose in one month. This is a healthy and maintainable loss that, if done according to the Power Foods Lifestyle™, you can be assured this is body fat loss only—not water or muscle tissue.

3. Think about three behaviors that you'll need to change in order for you to accomplish that goal. One behavior should be based on nutrition, another on physical activity, and the last one on mental discipline.
   - Example: Stop eating junk food.
   - Example: Work out more.
   - Example: Stop calling myself fat.

4. Think about two emotional triggers or obstacles that may prevent you from changing each of the three behaviors. These should be statements of fact that reflect your personal tendencies and current habits.
   - Example: Junk food in the pantry is easily accessible.
   - Example: Skipping meals because I'm too busy.
   - Example: Too tired or busy to work out after a long day at work.
   - Example: Not having a plan when I do a workout so I tend to wander and feel unproductive.
   - Example: Every time I look in the mirror I pinch my fat.
   - Example: Every time I see a fit person I mentally tell myself how fat I am.

5. Now that you have identified your emotional triggers and obstacles, identify how you can prevent each item you listed from happening, or reprogram what happens in your mind when they do. Include the phrase "I will" in your statement. This reaffirms to you that you are planning to make a change by committing yourself to your plan.

- Example: Junk food in the pantry is easily accessible.

I will throw out all the junk food and stop buying it.

- Example: Skipping meals because I'm too busy.

I will fuel myself regularly with 6 meals per day.

- Example: Getting too busy or tired to go to the gym after work.

I will wake up an hour earlier to go to the gym.

- Example: Not having a plan when I do exercise so I justify a lazy workout.

I will write a weekly or daily plan the night before.

- Example: Every time I look in the mirror I pinch my fat.

Every time I look in the mirror, I will tell myself something I like about myself.

- Example: Every time I see a fit person I mentally tell myself how fat I am.

Every time I see a fit person, I will tell myself that I'm doing the things I need to in order to improve myself.

6. Create a way to be accountable for your new efforts in changing your behavior. Accountability is crucial to your success. Life can become far too busy for us to stay focused for very long. If we don't have a simple reporting method, we will forget our goals, our efforts, and then find ourselves unhappy for lack of progress in what we truly desire. Some of my favorite methods for daily accountability include the following:

- A chart on my closet with gold stars to stick on for days I have done well.
- Adding an all-day event of COMPLETE to my Google Calendar on days I have done well.
- Drop a dollar bill into a jar for every day I have done well. At the end of the month, I can use the money to buy a reward like a new article of clothing.

7. Lastly, learn how to phrase these behaviors in the correct way.

- Write them in the present tense.
- Always write your goals in a positive tense.
- Use action verbs.
- Keep your goal very clear and concise.
- Include an end date in your goal.

Words, and the way you use them, are critical in helping you view your goals with the right mindset. Be sure to follow these suggestions for the best results in your goal-setting. Remember the most important reason for focusing on goals: you will see results much faster as you break them down, write them down, think about them, and become accountable to them.

Below is an example of how your monthly goal chart might appear based on the instructions I provided earlier.

My Monthly Goal

I will weigh 170 lb. on December 14.

My 6 Behaviors of Accountability

1. I shop for and keep only healthy foods in my pantry.

2. I fuel myself regularly with six smaller meals per day.

3. I wake up at 5 a.m. to go to the gym before work on weekdays.

4. I spend a few minutes each night to plan my workout for the following day.

5. I tell myself something I like about myself every time I look in the mirror.

6. Whenever I see someone with a body I admire, I tell myself that I'm doing the things I need to improve myself.

4

Macronutrients

M ainstream marketing of dieting and weight loss products would have
you believe something absurd—that your body's health and weight are
completely based on the calories-in and calories-out mentality. This belief means
you are thinking of your body as a checking account, that making a "deposit" of
eating too many calories will result in a greater balance, or "weight gain," while
making a "withdrawal" of eating fewer calories or exercising more than normal will
result in a negative balance, or "weight loss." While on a functional level these
principles may arguably be true, there are many more factors to consider. The body is
far more complicated than that.

Hormones, lean body mass, resting metabolic rate, workout structure,
workout intensity, workout timing, meal timing, digestive enzymes, and your genetic
coding are all factors that differ from person to person. Simply reducing the number of
calories you eat in a day may or may not result in weight loss.

Have you heard the term "skinny-fat?" I really despise the word fat (I
encourage you to replace this word with fluffy—yes, laugh all you want, but this is a
game-changer over time to stop calling yourself fat); however, the term 'skinny-fat'
best describes what happens when a person loses weight by cutting calories without
applying a strategy to maintain or even build lean muscle mass. Despite being thin,
there is still a great deal of body fat on a "skinny-fat" person's body. There is nothing
inherently wrong with this look, so long as your body fat falls in a healthy range.*

The principles of the PFL will enhance your ability to sculpt your body
on a muscular level (if that is your desire and you're putting in the work at the
gym), all while chiseling the fat off your frame. In the first edition of this book, I
wrote that the PFL will also "promote a healthier system overall." At this point in

revising the book, however, it's amazing to me how many *additional* health factors are being treated and improved through the PFL and its adaptations by my team of Body Buddies coaches. The demographics of people finding incredible results include those with type I and type II diabetes, high cholesterol, high triglycerides, PCOS, insulin resistance, hypoglycemia, hyperglycemia, metabolic syndrome—even pregnancy (see my book *Power Foods for Two: A Lifestyle for the Pregnant Woman*). I have been blessed to work with those who experience anorexia, bulimia, or binge-eating disorder, and seen incredible changes happen in people's minds, behaviors, and consequently their bodies.

How are all of these amazing results occurring? By focusing on macronutrient portions, combinations, and distribution, which are the most important principles of the PFL. As you learn about them and their roles in your body, you will begin to experience some "a-ha" moments as you begin to better understand principles of nutritional science. You will recognize how simple principles unite to produce results in your body.

While understanding macronutrients is important, they are not enough on their own. You shouldn't neglect the micronutrients that fuel every one of your bodily processes. This is where I've done the hard work for you—the Power Foods I recommend that you eat the majority of the time are packed with micronutrients that will help your body function better on the cellular level, while the balance of macronutrients will help control the shape of your body aesthetically.

What in the world are macronutrients and micronutrients anyway? Let's break down the words:

Macro = big

Micro = small

Nutrient = nourishment

---

[1] World Health Organization 2013

When we talk about *macronutrients* (let's call them "macros" for short), we're talking about "big nutrients." The big nutrients in your food are known for providing your body with energy. There are three, and you should know them backward and forward:

1. Protein
2. Carbohydrate
3. Fat

When we talk about *micronutrients* (let's call them "micros" for short), we are talking about "small nutrients." The small nutrients in your food are known for providing your body with vitamins and minerals. These include, but are not limited to, the following:

1. Vitamin A
2. Vitamin B1
3. Vitamin B12
4. Vitamin B6
5. Calcium
6. Chromium
7. Vitamin C
8. Vitamin D
9. Vitamin E
10. Folate
11. Iodine
12. Iron
13. Vitamin K
14. Magnesium
15. Selenium
16. Thiamin
17. Zinc

What's Behind the Calories?

All calories are not created equally: consuming an ice cream sandwich will not have the same impact in your body as eating a small piece of chicken and green leaf lettuce, despite each of these food items containing 150 calories. You need to look beyond manufacturer labeling and advertising to make better health choices.

Marketers sure do a good job of enticing you to buy their products by playing to your desires for lower calories and weight loss, don't they? With a solid understanding of why those supposedly "healthy" and "weight-loss promoting" foods aren't actually helping you lose weight, you will be able to make strategic decisions and reach the results you are working towards on the inside and outside.

Each of the macronutrients have been scientifically proven to provide your body with approximate numbers of calories (let's remember that science hardly ever comes to round numbers, but these whole numbers are easier to use than a big long decimal):

Protein provides 4 calories per gram.
Carbohydrate provides 4 calories per gram.
Fat provides 9 calories per gram.

Notice how one gram of both protein and carbohydrate contributes 4 calories, while fat contributes 9 calories. Now, if you're in the mindset that total calories is of utmost importance, I hope you don't get your panties in a bundle over fat flaunting 9 calories per gram—this doesn't make fat bad and something to avoid. It simply means that you need to understand its composition, respect it through the types of fat you eat, and utilize strategies to cause dietary fats to aid you in your goals. We will talk more about fat in Chapter Seven (get excited, it will rock your world!)

Identifying Macronutrients and Peak Ranges

Take a look at the nutrition label as an example to find where macros are located on every FDA-approved food product.

Now that you know where to find each of the numbers, let's talk about what they mean. I know this information can be overwhelming at first, but do your best to understand the next section. It's very important training for you to learn how to identify foods on your own so that you can easily apply principles of the PFL for the rest of your life.

To qualify as a power food, one macronutrient number needs to far exceed the other two. For instance, carbohydrates need to hit a "peak range," or an appropriate range for a meal while protein and fat are far below their peak ranges. Aiming to hit a peak range for each type of meal is important as you balance your meals. You will be able to decide if a food has adequate grams of protein, carbohydrate, or fat to properly fuel your body and fulfill a P, C, or F in a meal.

Below are my recommended peak ranges per meal for generally healthy and active adults.[2] Please remember these ranges are for promoting slow and steady fat loss; we will cover maintenance in a later chapter.

Protein: 15-30 grams
Carbohydrate: 20-30 grams
Fat: 8-12 grams

When one of a food's macronutrient grams lands in a peak range, you can use it strategically for a Power Foods meal. There are many foods that will easily fall in the peak range of two or even all three macro categories. The difficult part is in finding a food that hits only one of the three peaks, while the other two stay very minimal in their numbers. The overwhelming majority of foods that fit the Power Foods description are naturally-occurring foods. They are not processed in a factory. Foods that fit the description of power foods can be called power proteins, power carbohydrates, and power fats. There may be many "healthy" foods that do not qualify as a power food.

Nutrition Facts

Serving Size 1 cup (110g)
Servings Per Container About 6

Amount Per Serving

Calories 200   Calories from Fat 30

                                                    % Daily Value*

Total Fat 4g	**11%**
Saturated Fat 3g	**16%**
Trans Fat 0g	
Cholesterol 4mg	**2%**
Sodium 150mg	**13%**
Total Carbohydrate 10g	**10%**
Dietary Fiber 3g	**14%**
Sugars 2g	
Protein 6g	

Vitamin A	7%
Vitamin C	15%
Calcium	20%
Iron	32%

* Percent Daily Values are based on a 2,000 calorie diet. Your daily value may be higher or lower depending on your calorie needs.

		Calories:	2,000	2,500
Total Fat		Less than	55g	75g
Saturated Fat		Less than	10g	12g
Cholesterol		Less than	1,500mg	1,700mg
Total Carbohydrate			250mg	300mg
Dietary Fiber			22mg	31mg

1. Chicken breast has a high protein content with 26 grams per 4 ounces, but a very low content of carbohydrates and fat (less than 1-2 grams of both per 4-ounce serving). Because the protein number far exceeds the grams of fat and carbohydrates, chicken breast is a power food under the category of protein.

*Protein: 26 grams (falls in the peak range for protein)
Carbohydrate: <1 gram (does not fall in the peak range for carbohydrate)
Fat: 2 grams (does not fall in the peak range for fat)

---

[2] Please keep in mind that it is very difficult to provide ranges that will fit every person's gender, genetic makeup, metabolism, etc. If you are interested in better understanding the specific ranges with analysis of your current eating habits, blood type, body type, and athletic involvement, please visit the Body Buddies Coaching page at www.body-buddies.com.

In contrast, ham has a moderately high protein content with 18 grams per 4 ounces, low carbohydrate content of 2 grams, but a high content of fat with 10 grams per 4 ounces. Ham hit two of the macronutrient peaks, instead of one. Therefore, ham is not a power food.

*Protein: 18 grams (falls just under the peak range for protein)
Carbohydrate: 2 grams (does not fall in the peak range for carbohydrates)
*Fat: 10 grams (falls in the peak range for fats)

2. Oats have high carbohydrate content (roughly 30 grams per ½ cup) in proportion to a lower protein content of 5 grams and lower fat content of 3 grams per ½ cup. This makes oats a power food under the category of carbohydrate. (Let's keep in mind that power carbohydrates don't need a low protein content. Grains like quinoa and legumes like black/ kidney beans have slightly higher protein— though still far below a peak range. This doesn't take away from the fact that they are a power carb—the protein content is simply a bonus.)

Protein: 5 grams (does not fall in the peak range for protein)
*Carbohydrate: 30 grams (falls in the peak range for carbohydrates)
Fat: 3 grams (does not fall in the peak range for fats)

In contrast, a large croissant has a low protein content of 7 grams with a higher carbohydrate content of 25 grams and a higher fat content of 6 grams. Croissants hit just below two of the macronutrient peaks, instead of one. Therefore, croissants are not a power food.

Protein: 7 grams (does not fall in the peak range for protein)
*Carbohydrate: 25 grams (falls in the peak range for carbohydrates)
*Fat: 6 grams (falls just below the peak range for fats)

3. Almonds have a high fat content of 7 grams per ½ ounce in proportion to lower content of protein (3 grams) and carbs (3 grams) per ½ ounce. Don't forget that fat contains 9 calories per gram, so that seemingly small number of 8 grams has actually more energy than you think. Carbohydrates and protein have 4 calories per gram, so naturally, you can consume more volume for the same energy. This fact may direct you to eating mostly protein and carbohydrates, which is understandable logic, but I need you to know that

is flawed logic. Keep in mind that your body needs fats, so the strategic use of power food fats is essential. As the types of fat in almonds are primarily monounsaturated and polyunsaturated fats, almonds are a power foods under the category of fat.

Protein: 3 grams (does not fall in the peak range for protein)
Carbohydrate: 3 grams (does not fall in the peak range for carbohydrates)
*Fat: 7 grams (falls just under the peak range for fats)

In contrast, margarine has a high fat content of 11 grams per Tablespoon in proportion to lower content of protein (<1 gram) and carbohydrate (0 grams). While it may appear that margarine is a Power Food under the category of fat, it is not. This is because the primary ingredients in margarine include safflower, soybean, rapeseed, or cottonseed oil—oils known for their Trans fat content. (We will discuss healthy oils in a later chapter.) Therefore, margarine is not a power food while butter is.

Protein: <1 gram (does not fall in the peak range for protein)
Carbohydrate: 0 grams (does not fall in the peak range for carbohydrates)
*Fat: 11 grams (falls in the peak range for fats)

Macronutrient balancing is a healthful way to eat and train the cells in your body to function as they were designed, leading to loss of stubborn body fat. You should no longer solely count calories as your method of gauging success in losing body fat. Remember to think of preserving the environment of your body more than thinking of it as a bank account. While total calories are important, their importance is secondary to the composition and combination of nutrients of which the calories are comprised.

Common Myths about Calories

Here are two simple principles I would like you to understand:

1. Weight loss and weight gain are dependent on burning more, or less, than the number of calories you consume. If you take in more calories than your body burns in a day, you may gain weight. If you take in fewer calories than your body burns in a day, you may lose weight. There are exceptions to every rule due to hormones and metabolic processes, but this is generally true for most people.

2. Every calorie is not created equally. The quality of the nutrients behind the calories, along with their combination to create a fat-burning and nutrient-absorbing environment, is what makes the greatest difference in your health and body shape.

How many times have you meticulously counted calories and made sure to hit your goal for daily totals on the dot? Does this method drive you nuts? Did you find it maintainable? Did you find it to suck away so much of your focus and time?

Perhaps you fall on the other side of the spectrum and have never counted a calorie in your life. This whole "paying attention to what you eat" thing may be super new to you (and quite annoying, am I right?). No matter which mentality you claim, I hope you will leave this next section with a different mentality, the desire to begin retraining your mind because of what you learn.

For over ten years, calorie-counting ran my life. Whether it was a little notebook full of hand-written numbers that I carried everywhere, an entry on my phone, or a simple mental calculation every time I ate, I was obsessed. Full-blown obsessed. I grew fixated on the foods that I could and couldn't eat. I labeled foods as 'good' and 'bad' due to their caloric content. I constantly solved math equations to track how many calories I had eaten and compared them to the calories the cardio machines told me I'd burned. I couldn't focus on the more important things in life because I was preoccupied with controlling the food that went into my body.

Over the past few years, I have learned to change my thought patterns and attitude toward calories. I realize I was making some very big mistakes in being so meticulous. I didn't yet understand the other issues that made a difference. Perhaps *you* don't know this yet either.

Have you ever found yourself thinking along these lines?
- I should "save up" my calories so I can eat a bigger meal later in the day.
- Eating sugar-free, low-fat, and non-fat foods will help me reach my goals.
- I should look for the foods that are lowest in calories so I can eat more food today.

With a little more information on why this way of thinking isn't ideal, I hope you will see there are better ways to approach food. These common approaches to fat **loss and dieting** may actually be slowing your progress.
Flawed Logic: I should "save up" my calories so I can eat a bigger meal later in the day.

Skimping on food earlier in the day slows your metabolism instead of keeping it going when you can burn the most calories. After all, food is fuel. If you don't put fuel in a car, it's not going to move very quickly, right? It's the same thing with your body. Think of your metabolism as the entire combination of all of your bodily processes. The "higher" your metabolism, the more efficient the chemical processes are in your body. A "sluggish metabolism" is a slower, less efficient functioning of chemical processes.

When you don't eat much, you're not getting as many nutrients and energy during the prime energy-burning part of your day, which is between breakfast and lunch. *Notice how I didn't give times since breakfast and lunch times differ from person to person. Your body clock is different than others so be sure to review the chapter on meal timing.* Your body senses the lack of nourishment, resulting in a significant slowing of your metabolism to preserve energy. When you finally eat your big meal, your blood sugar levels rapidly rise from their lowered state where they had been resting due to your lack of eating. Your body cannot use fat for fuel when your blood sugar rises. When you eat highly-processed carbs or sugar (arguably the same thing) an insulin spike is produced which turns off your fat-burning. "For how long?" I am often asked. Depending on the amount and types of food you consume, this could be anywhere from a 2–24 hour window. The release of insulin from your pancreas signals your body to transport and store the nutrients that remain in your blood stream after absorbing and transporting the nutrients it actively needs. Storage is never a good thing if you are trying to shed excess body fat. This is why your body's environment and the stability of your blood sugar must be preserved.

If the insulin spike isn't bad enough, the real problem is that the spike happens so close to your bedtime. In addition to knocking your body out of its fat-burning environment, eating a larger meal later in the day results in excess calories that need to go through the digestion and absorption process while you sleep. The odds are that your body is going to absorb the excess energy and pull it into adipose (fat) tissue for storage rather than burn through them. Regardless of how many calories you "saved" or "burned" earlier in the day, your body does not become that bank account that sits there and calculates the difference. Everything is about the environment of the body.

Flawed Logic: Eating sugar-free, low-fat, and non-fat foods will help me reach my goals.

This includes foods with labels that read as follows:

- Low-fat
- Fat-Free
- Reduced Fat
- Sugar-Free
- Reduced Calories
- Diet

These types of phrases present you with a false reality—that the food inside the packaging is a better choice than its alternative. As a result, you may feel as though the food or beverages are safe to consume and will actually help you reach your goals. But watch out—any unnatural food that has been chemically processed to change its composition will also alter your body's chemicals and hormones, thus affecting the environment that we have discussed.

Keeping in mind that all foods are chemical compounds, let's be clear that we are talking about artificial, man-made chemicals. These types of chemicals don't just magically pass through your body without influencing something along the way. Reduced fat or fat-free foods have been chemically altered in a factory, packed with preservatives and additives to make up for the lack of the food's normal chemical structure.

Artificial sweeteners are often hundreds of times sweeter than normal sugar, which desensitizes you to a natural taste. Eventually, the consumption of artificial sweeteners will promote weight gain, not fat loss, as you need more and more to satisfy your craving for a sweet taste. These foods also lack vital nutrients and will cause you to pack on more pounds as the additives are all highly addictive. All of these awesome-looking reduced calorie and low-fat foods are not magic, they're simply deceptive. They will not help you reach your goals for the long-term.

Flawed Logic: I should look for the foods that are lowest in calories so I can eat more food today.

So what if the food (or food-like product) has low calories? What nutrients compose those calories? Are they a well-balanced mix of important, energy-yielding macronutrients? How much sugar is in each serving? How many naturally-occurring vitamins and minerals are in the food? How much artificial sweetener is in the food? Hold onto these questions because we will cover them later.

Does your food label say "enriched," meaning the factory added nutrients into the food artificially? If your food product comes in a factory-labeled container or box and states it has low calories, chances are the food-like substance contains few vital nutrients that occur naturally, and that the macronutrients are not going to be balanced or strategically designed to help you achieve a healthier body shape.

I know it can be very discouraging to look around the grocery store with your growing knowledge from this book and realize just how few foods actually fall in the category of power foods. You want foods that are "fun" and "tasty," yet I will tell you this: justification in eating low calorie, reduced fat, or diet foods will not get you to faster results—only to a growing frustration as time passes. Please take what I'm saying at face value and decide to be a responsible person who is educated and takes control over your eating behavior. You can do this!

Conclusion

From here on out, please stop counting calories. Instead, focus on eating appropriate portion sizes of power foods. We will cover portions in a later chapter, so keep reading. There is so much to learn! As your focus on calories decreases and you focus, instead, on energy balance of power foods, your body will slowly begin to change. You will begin to understand how powerful your body can feel. You probably have no idea just how much you've been living below your body's potential. I can't wait for you to experience it!

Be patient with yourself and the inevitable learning curve as you apply what you have learned. Remember, it takes a good two to three weeks to truly become immersed in new material or habits. I promise that your new healthy lifestyle will not take as much effort in the future; during the first few weeks, however, you do need to invest the time to learn and adapt.

The Power Foods Lifestyle isn't supposed to be the easy quick-fix approach that you fall in love with immediately. The PFL created itself. I was simply given the blessing of understanding it and am making my best efforts to explain it in simple terms you can understand and apply. Please invest some time in yourself to truly think about and apply the principles you are learning. You will intensify your learning by becoming an avid listener of the Body Buddies Podcast, which you can find on iTunes (iPhone), Stitcher Radio (Android), or directly on www.body-buddies.com.

Start by looking in your fridge and pantry for Power Foods. Can you easily find a non-Power Food? If so, go ahead and throw it out or give it away.

5

Protein

P rotein is powerful, pure and simple. This macronutrient provides strength for every cell and structure in your body whether it's muscle, bone, organ, tendon, or ligament. It helps all of your organs function properly, and facilitates blood transport and clotting of your blood when you cut yourself.

Your body contains thousands of different proteins, each with a specific function determined by its unique shape. Some act as enzymes, speeding up chemical reactions. Others act as hormones, which are like messengers for chemicals in your body. Antibodies made of protein protect you from foreign substances. Proteins maintain fluid balance by pumping molecules across cell membranes and attracting water. They maintain the acid and base balance of your body fluids by taking up, or giving off hydrogen ions as needed. Finally, proteins transport many key substances such as oxygen, vitamins, and minerals to target cells throughout your body.

Okay, blah, blah, blah, I know, it can be really boring to read these kinds of scientific facts and your eyes are glazing over. But here's the truth, plain and simple. Your body needs protein in every single meal. It's important for many different reasons, but some I'd like you to remember include these three:

1. Protein will help you feel fuller longer.

2. Protein will decrease your sugar cravings.

3. Protein will help keep your insulin from spiking too high—I like to call this "anchoring."

How Much Protein?

The Food and Drug Administration frequently changes the RDA (Recommended Daily Allowance) for macronutrients. The current recommendation for protein is 20-25% of your daily calories, assuming a 2,000 calorie diet. Well, Body Buds, as you follow the Power Foods Lifestyle, you are actually going to be getting 35-40%[3] of your calories from protein, assuming a 1,500 calorie intake. That's a range of 130-150 grams for an average active adult. Why is this, and why would it go against the RDA?

In nearly every clinical study performed, protein appears to make a stronger contribution to feeling satisfied after eating a meal than fats or carbohydrates. Most people tend to control the portions of their lunch meal more if they eat protein with breakfast than those who don't.

If you don't eat any more calories than usual, increasing the amount of protein you consume will help decrease the number of carbohydrates you put in your body. As you will learn in the next chapter, carbs are the number one insulin-producing macronutrient when over-consumed (remember that insulin is a storage hormone). Every study I have ever read about body fat loss, muscle toning, and improved health has included a higher recommended protein intake than the average American currently eats.

Not only do multiple studies show the health benefits in higher protein intake, but I have lived this lifestyle for the past three years and have experienced the difference. Each of my clients, and all those who have already changed their bodies and lifestyles using the PFL, can see the difference in their body as well. Higher protein intake contributes to losing unwanted body fat as it aids metabolic processing and decreases consumption of carbohydrates, ultimately stabilizing your blood sugar. This is particularly an important principle for older adults to implement as muscle wasting happens as you age.

Here are the power protein sources for the Power Foods Lifestyle:

- Chicken Breast/Tenders
- Egg Whites
- Ground Turkey (94% + learn, >6% fat)
- Lean Pork
- Lean Ground Beef (90% + lean, >10% fat)
- Orange Roughy
- Cottage Cheese (2% fat)
- Elk
- Halibut
- Lean Sirloin Steak
- Mahi Mahi
- Plain Greek Yogurt (2% fat)

---

[3] Exceptions always apply. Our team of coaches work to help individuals find the right protein intake for their body, age, gender, and goals.

- Protein Powder
- Salmon
- Swai Filet
- Tofu
- Tuna (packed in water)

- Red Snapper
- Shrimp
- Tilapia
- Turkey Breast

Below is a list of things to keep in mind when choosing these protein sources:

Cottage Cheese, Plain Greek Yogurt

Use 2% cottage cheese and plain Greek yogurt as opposed to fat-free. The less processing a food product encounters, the better it is for your body on a chemical level. Many studies have found that people who eat regular-fat dairy have lower risks of cardiovascular disease and developing diabetes than those with lower levels of dairy fat. These vitamins are tough to get in the diet from other sources. While plain Greek yogurt is getting more difficult to find in grocery stores, remember that it's worth the hunt! Although cottage cheese and plain Greek yogurt have residual grams of carbs and fats in them, we still consider them to be power foods for protein. Dairy fat is a good source of fat-soluble vitamins like retinol and vitamin K2.

Egg Whites

The most bioavailable (ready for your muscle tissue to utilize immediately) egg proteins are in raw egg whites or soft poached eggs that have not yet reached 160 degrees. The harder cooked your egg white, the more protein is denatured making the protein slower digesting. By the way, the chance of you getting salmonella from raw egg whites is 1 in 10,000 for regular eggs and 1 in 20,000 for free-range eggs. Egg-based liquid protein (like MuscleEgg® or Egg Whites International®) are excellent as well.

Lean Sirloin Steak, Lean Ground Beef (90% + lean, >10% fat)

Red meat is known for its saturated fat, which contrary to popular belief, is not entirely the bad guy. Instead, look at saturated fat and seek to keep it lower in ratio to monounsaturated and polyunsaturated fats— heart-healthy fats. As the saturated fat may reach close to the peak range for fat, you can see that adding a carb (like a baked potato) or a fat (like avocado) might overdo the energy balance of the meal. Due to its higher fat content, red meat is best eaten with vegetables only in a PV(F is assumed). Incorporate lots of leafy greens into the veggies with red meat to aid in digestion.

Red meat is actually very beneficial for your body, despite popular belief. It's a rich source of vitamin B12; deficiencies of this vitamin can play a role in cardiovascular disease, infertility, and mental illness. Red meat contributes heme iron, which helps your body absorb non-heme iron, a critical part of an expecting mother's nutritional intake. Thyroid function is best when red meat is a moderate part of your nutritional intake as it aids in synthesis of thyroid hormones. Due to commercial meat being packed with antibiotics and hormones, organic and grass-fed beef is the safest form to eat.

Though I definitely don't recommend consuming it every day, 1-3 servings per week is a nutritionally-sound amount. Some of the leanest cuts of red meat to look for include the following:

1. Eye Round Roast
2. Sirloin Tip Side Steak
3. Top Round Roast and Steak
4. Bottom Round Roast and Steak
5. Top Sirloin Steak

Remember: these aren't 12 oz. steaks I'm talking about. With a peak range of 15-30 grams per protein serving, you should be putting only 3-6 oz. of meat on your plate per serving. You can easily eyeball a typical serving size of an animal protein—it is the equivalent size of a deck of playing cards.

Halibut, Mahi Mahi, Orange Roughy, Red Snapper, Salmon, Shrimp, Swai Filet, Tilapia, Tuna (packed in water)

Wild-caught and farm-raised fish are nearly identical in terms of calories, protein, and most nutrients. You may wonder if farmed fish are genetically modified. No, not currently in the United States. Currently, the United States regulations prohibit the use of hormones or antibiotics to promote growth in farmed fish, so that shouldn't be a concern. The biggest difference between wild-caught and farm-raised fish is the levels of potentially carcinogenic chemicals, in particular PCBs.

Protein Myths

• Too much protein will make you bulky

This is a fear-based statement and scientifically flawed on all levels. I hear this concern a lot, especially from women. Though I would like to validate your fears as I, too, used to have this fear when I was a newbie to competitive training and fitness nutrition, my former fears were completely founded on hearsay instead of science. Now that I have years of experience of training my body and so many others' bodies as well, I feel confident in telling you that, yes, eating higher amounts of protein (about 1 ounce per pound of goal body weight) will give you the foundation to put on some muscle if you work hard in the gym. If you are not putting in the work to break down and rebuild your muscle fibers, protein will contribute nothing more than another source of energy for your body. Dietary intake alone cannot shape your physique and synthesize new lean muscle tissue. You must be training hard enough to build muscle.

The feeling of puffiness you get after lifting is not due to instant gains in muscle (though I sure wish that were the case). This physical response is an extracellular swelling as you have successfully disturbed the fluid balance of your body, along with the stress hormone cortisol, resulting in your body retaining water. Don't worry, it should subside after a few hours and as you fuel yourself with lean protein and power carbs—which are those low on the glycemic index.

- Heating up protein powder ruins the protein

Denaturation is a process by which the protein structure alters shape through external stress—in the case of cooking, that's usually by heat. Sure, heat will cause the protein coils to unwind and alter shape, but this doesn't change anything or damage it. Your body will absorb the same amino acids from the protein whether it's cooked or not. Your body is an amazing machine that takes the amino acid strands to form dietary protein that can be used in the cells.

- Peanut butter is a protein source

Sure, while there is protein in peanut butter, it is primarily a fat source with 8 grams of fat per tablespoon, and only 4 grams of protein. As a peak range of protein is 15-30 grams, you can see how deficient a mere 4 grams appears while the 8 grams falls beautifully in fat's peak range of 8-12 grams per meal. The protein content is simply a bonus in this primarily fat-based food.

- Cheese is a protein source

Cheese also has good amino acids (the building blocks of protein). However, the number of fat grams is simply too high for this to qualify as a power protein food. A power protein food must have very low carbohydrates and fats in comparison with its high protein content. Instead, we will count cheese as a power fat. The protein content is simply a bonus in this primarily fat-based food.

Protein as a Part of the Power Foods Lifestyle

Seek to eat a source of protein with every meal. Because you will be eating approximately six meals per day on the Power Foods Lifestyle (assuming you are sleeping 6-8 hours each night), this means you will be eating a protein source six times per day. Eating protein-based foods is a very consistent and predictable part of your daily routine once you adapt to this lifestyle.

Does this meal have a good source of protein? This phrase should become a constant question in your mind as you eat your meals and gain experience with it as the foundation of every meal. Whether you are preparing your meals at home, dining out, or are on vacation, your awareness of protein content will have far-reaching impacts on your long-term health and body composition. You must have your protein to complete the meal, feel full, and be satisfied. If you are low in your protein intake, I can guarantee you that you will be hungry before your next meal and experience more sugar cravings as well.

Use these guidelines in identifying whether or not a food fulfills your protein requirement per meal. These ranges are per serving:

- Protein: 15-30 grams
- Carbs: <5 grams
- Fats: <2 grams
- Sugar: <5 grams
- Calories: <250

What about Milk?

I meet many people who believe that milk is a great source of protein, and even one of the healthiest foods for the human body as many claim it to be the "best source of calcium." While I used to believe this common thread of what was thought to be fact, recent studies have changed my mind. In studies as early as 1994, milk consumption was found not only to lack prevention of fractures in adult women,[4] but to increase risk factors for hip fractures in the elderly.[5]

While milk is healthy and provides nutrients and vitamins, it does not qualify as a power food. While one cup of milk contains a moderate number of 8 grams of protein, it is not in the range that would make it a power protein. Additionally, there are approximately 12 grams of sugar in every cup of milk—no

---

[4] Feskanich D, Willett WC, Stampfer MJ, Colditz GA. Milk, dietary calcium, and bone fractures in women: a 12-year prospective study. American Journal of Public Health. 1997
[5] *"Case Control Study of Risk Factors for Hip Fractures in the Elderly."* American Journal of Epidemiology. Vol. 139, No. 5, 1994.

matter if it's skim or full-fat. Although this is lactose, a naturally-occurring sugar that doesn't necessarily produce a large insulin effect, many studies show enough gastrointestinal distress from large populations of milk-drinkers for me to curtail milk from our power foods list.

Now, let's get something straight: I am not condemning milk. I grew up in a household of nine people (yep, seven kids, all two years apart) that went through one gallon of 2% milk every day. We loved milk and it was something we regularly drank. Every one of us is healthy, fit, active, and have healthy habits thanks to our parents. So why did I make the switch to unsweetened almond milk, coconut milk, cashew milk, coconut milk, and leave my 2% regular milk for my indulgences?

I tested how I felt after drinking milk for several weeks and alternated with non-dairy alternatives. During this time, I experienced increased cravings for sugar and carbs. This was enough for me to take my own body's intuition over a glycemic index number on a chart and make the switch for my leaning out phases and maintenance phases. Bulking phases (intentionally overfeeding for muscle gains), however, are when I employ milk regularly with my protein shakes.

If you're concerned about not getting enough calcium by cutting out milk, rest assured. When you are eating as many leafy greens as the Power Foods Lifestyle promotes, you will be getting great sources of calcium constantly. I regularly take a calcium supplement as all women should, and all men might consider, in my recommendation. Tofu is also a great source of calcium and is on our power protein list.

Does all of this information mean you shouldn't drink milk? Not necessarily. You should do what feels right to you and learn your own body intuition instead of simply blindly following what I, or anyone else for that matter, tells you. This is your new lifestyle. I don't think there needs to be an all-or-nothing line—there's a great way to balance using milk in your lifestyle, like post-workout. Trust yourself enough to take into consideration all of the facts, and make an appropriate decision for yourself. Again, that's what the PFL is all about. Implementing new habits in your lifestyle due to education.

Vegans and Vegetarians

Protein comes in many different types of foods. In fact, you will most likely find a few grams of protein in nearly every food you eat. However, the majority of foods that meet power protein peak ranges come from animal and dairy sources. While many people are okay with these animal sources, there are large populations that for one reason or another, choose to abstain from eating these types of foods.

If you aren't sure the difference between Veganism and Vegetarianism, let's do a quick review:

Vegans: abstain from the use of animal products
Octo-lacto Vegans: abstain from red meat and poultry, but still consume eggs, dairy, and other animal-derived substances.
Vegetarians: abstain from consuming meat (red meat, poultry, seafood, and flesh of any other animal).

All plants (beans, vegetable, and grains) have the essential amino acids your body needs. Of course, some of these plant-based foods might have less protein than others, but each food provides adequate protein for general health. Be warned, however, that it's an arduous task to get a "high" protein intake while following a Vegan lifestyle, and you may find yourself overcompensating in other areas (carbohydrates and fats).

In order to reach the level of protein to fit your meal requirements, you would need to increase the portion size of your non-animal protein sources. Doing so will not only increase your caloric intake, but the number of carbs and/or fat in that meal. This will require you to adjust the portion, if not completely eliminate, the other macronutrient requirement from that particular meal—usually this is the carbohydrate source. For instance, let's look at quinoa. This is one of the highest protein-containing plant-based foods.

1/2 c. cooked quinoa

- Protein: 6 grams
- Carbs: 27 grams
- Fat: 3 grams
- Calories: 160

As you can see, quinoa is primarily a carbohydrate as 27 is in the peak range for a carbohydrate serving. With only 6 grams of protein, you would need approximately 4 servings to reach the protein intake goal for one meal. This would require you to eat 1.25 cups of quinoa, which would put you at 640 calories, 108 grams of carbohydrates, and 18 grams of fat. Quinoa doesn't seem like a power food for protein anymore, does it? That's because it isn't. While acknowledging that it is the highest protein-containing grain out there, we need to remember that this is a power carbohydrate source.

Let's Start Adapting

If you are a Vegan, there are some adaptations you will need to make to the PFL, the first of which will be protein powder. In each of the Power Foods Lifestyle recipes, I use a whey isolate powder, which is high in protein and very low (< 5 grams) in carbs. As whey protein is a product derived from cows, search for a Vegan protein that is lower in carbohydrates that you can substitute.

As animal protein composes the majority of the power protein column in the PFL, the structure of your meal combinations will change slightly. In working with many Vegans and Vegetarians, I found that the following basic structure is most conducive to meeting your aesthetic and health needs:

Meal 1: PVC
Meal 2: VCC
Meal 3: PVCC
Meal 4: VC
Meal 5: PVFF
Meal 6: PVF

Let's translate that into real food using our peak range portion sizes. Note: a capital letter represents a full peak range serving of that macronutrient, where a lower-case letter represents a half peak range serving. This meal plan will be for an Octo-Lacto Vegan.

Meal 1:	4 egg whites (P)
	½ bell pepper (V)
	¼ c. Grapenuts® cereal (C)
	½ c. unsweetened almond milk (not enough nutrients to be classified as anything)
	1/3 c. raspberries (c)
Meal 2:	½ c. cooked lentils (C)
	½ c. cooked black beans (C)
	10 baby carrots (V)
Meal 3:	½ c. cottage cheese (2%) (P)
	½ c. cooked kidney beans (C)

1 c. broccoli (V)
2 lightly salted plain rice cakes (C)

Meal 4: 1 Tbsp. natural peanut butter (F)
2 stalks celery (V)

Meal 5: 2 c. leafy greens (V)
1 Roma tomato (V)
2 hard-boiled eggs (PF)
12 raw almonds (F)

Meal 6: ½ c. plain Greek yogurt (2%) (P)
1 Tbsp. PB2® powder (not enough nutrients to
be classified as anything) *Powdered peanut butter is void of the oils,
so not classified as a fat like peanut butter.*
1/8 c. chopped raw walnuts (F)
½ med. Cucumber (V)

What will be most important in your personal strategy are these two items:

1. Pairing two complex carbohydrates together in a meal to keep total carb content from that PVC meal to 30-50 g.

2. Your carbohydrate intake will go later into the evening, so don't worry about that to make up for the calories unattained through regular protein intake. Initially, work on separating power carbs from power fats in meals. It may require some forethought and effort, but will soon become easier with practice.

Last but not least, please try not to substitute protein powder for more than two meals per day. As someone trying to live the PFL, it is important to get your nutrients and energy from whole foods for the majority of your meals.

Lactose Intolerance

If you are lactose intolerant, this means your body cannot easily digest lactose, which is a natural sugar found in milk and dairy products. Egg whites, whey protein, cheese, cottage cheese, and plain Greek yogurt are among the Power Foods you will need to exchange with other foods. You might also search health stores for lactose-free products that you can use regularly. You may find yourself using tofu or protein powder more often if you want to keep animal consumption to 2–3x per day (my typical recommendation).

Protein and your Workout

When you're eating protein at every meal, you're fueling your body for a beneficial workout by providing constant supplies of amino acids. Amino acids are the building blocks for protein synthesis—the construction of proteins that build new muscle tissues. Protein synthesis takes place after the workout, provided you have the right fuel, and allows your muscles to recover and grow stronger.

As you follow these principles, you will be able to contribute to building a stronger physique (as you engage in resistance training) and do so without being overly obsessive.

1. Make sure that one of your balanced meals falls approximately one hour before you **begin** your workout.

a. Combine your protein source with either a carb or a fat. You may learn very quickly that your body functions better with a PC (protein-carb) meal before a workout rather than a PF (protein-fat) combo meal. That's the fun of this lifestyle—figuring out which combos work best for your body.

b. I typically don't eat a veggie pre-workout but that's a personal preference. Your body might love a veggie pre-workout. Review the Meal Timing chapter which discusses timing of eating around a workout first thing in the morning.

2. Eat your next meal within 30-60 minutes following your workout.

a. It's best to choose a PVC meal (protein-veggie-carb) for a post-workout meal as the carbohydrates will help to replenish your glycogen (energy) supply. Increasing the portion of your power protein at this meal is also helpful to provide your body with the best nutrients to help your muscles heal and rebuild. If your workout comes right before bedtime, you may want to evaluate if fat loss or muscle protein synthesis is your higher goal. If it's the former, opt for a PVF meal over a PVC meal.

3. **Consider** drinking a protein shake within 30 minutes of finishing your workout.

a. If you are working to tone or build lean muscle tissue and putting in the training time and intensity to do so, consider having a post-workout shake so your body can absorb the protein more quickly. This will function as a P on its own, and is in addition to your regularly-timed balanced PVC or PVF meals. When your body is in a depleted state like after your workout, amino acids are able to be absorbed as new proteins and reach your muscles quicker. This aids in the refueling and rebuilding of your muscles.

The 30-60 minutes following your workout has a special name—the Anabolic Window. This is the time that your muscles need fuel to begin the process of repairing and rebuilding what you just worked to break down. Glycogen (stored energy in your muscles and your liver) needs to be replenished. You just did all of that work to break down your body, so don't deprive it of the fuel it needs in order to repair itself. This situation can be compared to going to the hairdresser with the intent of changing your hair color—the hairdresser sits you in front of the mirror and proceeds to put the color on your hair to make this change—but then never washes it out! Instead of completing the chemical work necessary to produce a vibrant and healthy change, the hair is damaged and cannot function or look as it did before. While this is an extreme analogy, the principle is the same. Breaking down your body without giving it nutrients to repair itself lacks wisdom and good strategy for changing your body composition for the better. Do your best to eliminate the mentality that you "just worked so hard to burn those calories" and you are "afraid to put more calories in your body." Knock it off. You're sending your body into starvation mode and turning your metabolism down severely by doing this.

While this is an important principle for many, keep in mind that when cutting body fat in an extremely controlled manner—like the way I train my natural bodybuilding competitors—a post-workout shake may or may not be used. What matters most is the timing of the nutrients (typically a PVC meal but can vary depending on the overall strategy of "building" versus "cutting") following the workout. I have trained many competitors who could not drink protein powder, and still prepared incredible physiques simply by having a PVC meal within the Anabolic Window. Choose what's best for you based on this information.

Protein Powders

Instead of saying "yes" or "no" to a product you wonder about using, I hope you will use the principles I teach to identify for yourself whether a product is conducive to you reaching your goals or not. There are many companies out there looking to make money from society's overwhelming desire for weight loss. Often, a new product is simply a replication of an already-existing product, just labeled differently. The supplement industry is still without regulation at the time of this book's revision. New products can pop up anywhere at any time as they are not subject to pre-market testing. Many nutritional supplements are not reviewed for their safety or effectiveness before hitting market shelves.

While I believe protein powder can be helpful for many people, I don't advocate that the supplement is for all demographics.

If you choose to be a consumer of protein powder, I encourage you to consider the following when purchasing:

1. Pay attention to the ratio of protein, carbs, fats, and sugar in a product you are looking into using. Ask yourself these questions:

a. Does the powder hit a protein peak range? (15–30 grams)

b. Does the powder hit a carbohydrate peak range? (15–30 grams)
If there are more than 5 grams of carbs per serving, keep in mind that you will need to account for the additional carbs as you follow the PFL recipes which utilize protein powder as an ingredient. Carbs in protein powder are neither good nor bad—this entirely depends on your goal and how you use the powder strategically around your workout, in combination with other foods, and the timing.

c. Does the powder hit a fat peak range? (8–12 grams)
If there is greater than 5 grams of fat, you might choose a different supplement as this is edging up toward a fat peak range.

d. Does the shake have enough calories to satisfy you for an entire meal? (Use this only if it's a meal replacement shake). Will you need to add food items to complete a PVC meal? The total calories in a meal that hits all macronutrient ranges for PVC or PVF should be between 200. Too few calories will result in feeling deprived, hungry, and contribute to losing control of your disciplined eating, being irritable and moody, and not following through with making your healthy eating a lifestyle.

2. How much taurine, glycine, glutamine, and creatine is in your choice of protein powder? Some companies have been caught adding extra amino acids to the mixture as it allows them to claim more dietary protein on the nutrition label for cheap. This is called amino acid spiking. Though legal, this is a deceptive practice to the uninformed consumer. You can beat these companies at their manipulative marketing game as you do the following when purchasing a powder:

a. Never buy a protein powder with creatine listed in the ingredient list.

b. Unless the full amino profile is disclosed, question those products with taurine, glycine, and glutamine in the listing, especially when these aminos come listed in a "protein blend." If these aminos come at the bottom of the ingredient list, you might not be too bamboozled by the shift in actual dietary protein composition.

High-quality protein powders with nutrition labels that fit PFL criteria don't come at a low cost. This is because they are the quality that your body needs and deserves. Any company will try to cut corners and make a less efficient product that they can offer for less money—it's a simple business principle. You will see the difference between protein powders that are on the grocery store shelves and protein powder found only in supplement stores or online. Always do what your budget dictates; I don't recommend going into debt for the sake of having the best protein out there. However, having a heightened awareness is key in helping you fuel your body in the best way possible.

Please be aware that a product that is endorsed or sponsored by a doctor with a medical degree is not automatically the best thing for you. Doctors need and want to make money as well, and with their endorsement comes a big fat pay check. Before looking into the credentials of any doctor and trusting their "knowledge," look into the ethical reputation of that doctor. Becoming an informed consumer and doing your own research is critical to your health in this world where business and ethics don't often mix. You may read more in-depth information about protein powders in the chapter on Supplements and Vitamins.

Conclusion

Protein is an essential macronutrient to help your body function properly. Regular consumption of 15-30 grams per meal will help your body avoid insulin spikes, provide the amino acids necessary to repair and rebuild damaged muscle tissue, and help you feel fuller longer. It will also help you better control your intake of carbohydrates and fats, which leads to a lower daily caloric intake. With every meal you construct, aim to include a power protein source. The more variety you include in your meals, the more your body will benefit from the varying nutrients.

Protein is a fundamental part of every meal in body reconstruction and maintenance.

6

Carbohydrates

M any companies are making incredible profits by manufacturing "low-carb" and "no-carb" products. Our society has grown desperate for these types of foods due to media's hyper-blogging, YouTube-ing, and talk show-ing the living daylights out of the notion that carbs are the bad guy. When millions of people want to lose weight and are equally misinformed about nutritional science, they end up buying these products in mass amounts. It's a brilliant business model to increase revenue, but very unfortunate for the people purchasing these products as it delivers no respite for their problem.

So let's get down to the nitty-gritty. Carbohydrates are not the bad guy; rather, they're wonderful! Your body loves and needs them! Your incredible body was designed to utilize this macronutrient to help it function properly. When you don't eat enough carbs, you may feel lethargic, irritable, and experience more significant cravings. This is your body sending you a signal that it needs fuel in the form of glucose (which comes primarily from carbs). Your central nervous system (CNS) functions primarily on the power of carbs.

When your brain stops receiving the glucose it needs to run efficiently, your neurons experience a crisis. As a result, you feel weak, spaced-out, tired, and unable to focus. The technical name of this low blood-sugar state is hypoglycemia. While your brain requires two times as much energy than other cells in your body, that doesn't mean you have license to eat muffins, breads, cookies, and chips all the time. We'll get to that, but first, let's talk some science so you can understand the basic concept of blood sugar. After all, I really need you to start thinking of your body as hosting an environment, and not working like a bank account. This shift in mindset will only happen as you open your mind to consider the science of blood sugar, insulin, and glucose.

I like to think of glycogen like a pearl necklace, as it's a way for your body to store little "pearls" of glucose. When the beads (glucose) are formed together for storage, they're stored in long chains (like a pearl necklace), which we call glycogen. This breakdown of carbohydrates to glucose begins in your mouth with your saliva. It then continues in your stomach, with gastric acid helping in the process. The broken-down carbohydrates are then ushered into your small intestine where absorption happens. At this point, the glucose molecules that aren't needed immediatley are transported through your body and stored in long branched chains of glycogen (think of the necklace again) in two storage sites: your liver and skeletal muscle.

When you don't have enough glycogen storage (due to lower than usual intake of carbs), you may lack energy in longer workouts. This is why people on low-carb diets often feel dizzy, weak, and tired. When your body needs energy—like during a workout or performing a physically-exerting task—your body breaks down the "pearl necklace" into the individual "pearls." Those pearls, or glucose, can then be used by your body to keep your blood glucose stable and give you energy. Your body can store anywhere from 200-500 milligrams of glycogen at one time.

The basic PFL structure utilizes carbohydrates strategically, accounting for approximately 35-40% of your daily caloric intake. However, it's important that you learn and master the strategies of utilizing carbohydrates. I have worked with many clients who have required more than, or less than, the recommendation I just made for average adults. Even while exceptions always apply, we need a dot on the map from which to start, so we'll continue onward with the 35-40% range.

Simple Carbs vs. Complex Carbs

When looking at a nutrition label, you will see a number of grams of carbohydrates listed. However, all carbohydrates are not created equally and won't have the same impact on your body, even if two different products' listed carbs are the same number.

Simple carbs are digested quickly and cause your insulin to be secreted, resulting in an insulin spike. Insulin triggers cells throughout your body to absorb glucose from your bloodstream, due to the raised blood sugar. Additionally, simple carbs contain fewer nutrients other than calories. They lack fiber and pass into the bloodstream rapidly, which is how they spike your insulin so quickly. An insulin spike is not conducive to body fat loss.

Examples:

- Sugars
- Syrups
- Fruit drinks
- Candy

- Honey
- Jams
- Sodas
- Cookies

Complex carbs digest slowly and are made of sugar molecules which are strung together. They help keep your blood sugar levels stable due to being rich in fiber, and contain many vitamins and minerals as they are generally found in whole plant foods.

Examples:

- Green vegetables
- Whole-grains

- Oatmeal
- Legumes

Utilizing the PFL principles and lingo (PVC/PVF meals) means you will be focused on eating complex carbs and staying away from simple carbs the majority of the time. There is a time and place to eat simple, highly-refined carb-based foods, but the key is to be wise and do your best every day for the situation you're in. I'd like you to understand the science behind the difference so you can best ascertain your body's need versus desire when making a choice. The carbs-based foods listed below are those I'd like you to regularly turn to when seeking to fulfill a C in your PVC meals:

- Apples
- Beans
- Bran Flakes
- Bread/Tortilla (Whole Wheat/Rye/Corn)
- Flour (Barley/Oat/Coconut/Wheat)
- Grapenuts®
- Oats
- Pumpkins
- Raspberries
- Rice (Long-grained Brown, Basmati, Wild)
- Whole Wheat Pasta

- Bananas
- Blueberries
- Chickpeas
- Couscous
- Grapefruit
- Lentils
- Oranges
- Quinoa
- Red Potatoes
- Strawberries
- Yams

Insulin: Our Friend, Our Enemy

Insulin is a hormone that originates in your pancreas. The secretion of insulin helps your body absorb and utilize the glucose you put in your body. Whenever you eat foods with carbohydrates, your blood sugar will rise. Your body senses this, and calls upon insulin to go out and do its job as a chemical messenger. Insulin then signals the little microvilli (finger-like projections) in your digestive tract to absorb the glucose, which will help the blood sugar levels regulate. As the glucose gets absorbed, your body will use anything that is actively needed for energy, then shuttle the rest into your liver and muscles for energy storage.

Remember talking about glycogen and the "pearl necklace" earlier? Up until this point, the process of what goes on when you eat carbs is part of the plan, no problem at all. That is, until the glucose senses a problem: if your liver and muscle are already full of glycogen, the excess glucose is at a dead-end. It can't be stored for energy storage so it is shuttled into a different form of storage—adipose tissue, which you know as body fat. This is why portion control of carbs-based foods is absolutely critical.

Insulin resistance is a problem that many people experience as well. Simply explained, this is when your body has called upon insulin to do its job so often and in such high amounts (you know all of those years of yo-yo dieting and sugar binges?) that a residue or film builds up and makes your body's response to insulin very weak. Insulin resistance leads to your body storing the energy from many of the foods you eat as visceral fat—the most dangerous form of fat as it surrounds the organs in your abdomen. If you would describe yourself as a "bigger-bellied" or "pear-shaped" person with more mass in your abdomen, I encourage you to pay strict attention to this opportunity to begin closely regulating the amount and types of carbs you eat. Through the PFL principles, I have watched many people help their bodies better respond to carbs and lose much of the dangerous visceral fat.

Carb Loading & Fatigue

The reason for carb loading is glycogen storage and providing fuel to athletes (particularly endurance athletes) to be broken down for energy in their workout with the help of insulin's counter-hormone, glucagon. Carb loading helps a person maximize their supply of glycogen, helping them workout harder and longer. Does this mean you should eat a gigantic spaghetti dinner the night before participating in an endurance sport? For most people, no. The storage available in your liver and muscles is limited, so if you over-consume carbs past your storage capacity, the excess will be stored as fat. There is a great deal of strategy in increasing your glycogen storage capacity over time that I have helped long-distance runners, bikers, and Ironmen athletes accomplish—but that is for another book or working with a Body Buddies Coach.

Like the gas tank in your car, you should only fill the tank to capacity. Avoid "topping off" or you will get "spill-over." Eating strategic portion sizes will give your brain and body enough glucose to function and have energy, while controlling the blood sugar response to further facilitate body fat loss. Regularly keep your carb intake to a strategic range (remember 20-30 grams per PVC meal for most active, healthy adults when trying to lose body fat.)

Have you ever hit that point, whether in your everyday life or during a workout, where you feel absolutely fatigued? This usually means you have depleted your glycogen storage and your body no longer has fast access to glucose to fuel itself. Sensing this, the hormone glucagon signals your body to begin breaking down stored fat as a way to get glucose for energy.

This is one of the reasons I recommend you do your cardio workout after resistance training if you are trying to lose body fat. When you follow this strategy, you are using your glycogen storage for energy to train hard and break down your muscles to sculpt and strengthen them. When your glycogen stores are depleted, performing aerobic cardio will primarily burn fat. If you haven't depleted your glycogen stores, it is more strategic for body fat loss to utilize high-intensity interval training (HIIT) which uses glucose for energy and provides a greater "afterburn." This is the amount of energy used in 24-48 hours post-exercise. Performing exercise at an aerobic threshold, which doesn't push you into the "huffin' puffin' gaspin' for air" threshold, will utilize fat for energy, but at a much lower caloric total over the course of 24 hours. This is why it's important for you to deplete your glycogen first if you plan to perform aerobic exercise at a lower heartrate than anaerobic exercise. I would love to talk more exercise science and how it relates to the Power Foods Lifestyle, but that's for another book, or for you to learn through the Body Buddies podcast and blogs.

Carbs and Fats' Relationship

This section covers one of the most important principles of the PFL and what separates the PFL from nearly every other method of eating out there. This is essential for you to understand in terms of strategy geared toward losing body fat. A maintenance or re-framing/bulking approach will differ, so please review the chapter on Maintenance and Miscellaneous Goals if you're in that phase of your lifestyle change and physique development.

Imagine you are going out for a nice evening with your significant other. You want to smell nice, so you spritz a little perfume or cologne onto your skin. Mmmmm, that's nice, you think. It smells wonderful and the scent wafts through the air. Do you then reach for a second bottle of a different scent of perfume or cologne? No—spraying a different scent on top of the first scent would completely dilute the original. It would also probably result in a pungent and overwhelming smell that would cause your significant other to wrinkle his or her nose.

This is exactly how you need to treat carbs and fats. I would like you to gain a keen awareness to keep these two energy macronutrients separated in your meals. On their own—combined with a source of protein and vegetables—carbs and fats are great. They each have their purpose and you need both carbs and fats in your daily food consumption for health and bodily function. But combining carbs and fats together in meals is not the most strategic way to eat for fat loss.

Here are several reasons why:

1. Your body utilizes both carbs and fats for energy, but they have different roles in your body. As carbs are your body's primary source of energy (remember how your brain uses glucose for fuel?), your body will always utilize the carbs for energy first if both carbs and fats are present in a meal (we are assuming full peak range portion sizes of both of these macronutrients). So if your body is using the carbs and experiences the rise in blood sugar, what does that leave the fat to do? The fats in the meal are first broken down into fatty acids, then packaged in bundles called triglycerides to be stored in your fat cells. All excess energy you consume will be stored in the body for later use, a.k.a. adipose tissue.

2. Simple awareness of carbs-based and fats-based foods will help you make wiser decisions and control your overall energy consumption. If you were at a work lunch and noted that there was lasagna (carbs in the noodles and fats in the cheese), breadsticks (carbs), a green salad (veggies), dressing (fats), and cookies (carbs), you could best strategize your overall macros consumption. As you see there are more carbs available than fats, you might wisely choose to go for a PVC meal over a PVF meal. This would be a strategic PFL-way of eating this meal:

- As the lasagna is both carbs and fats-based, choose a smaller portion, perhaps the circumference of your palm, so you don't get an overload of energy nutrients.
- Opt out of the cookie and the breadstick as you already have enough carbs in the lasagna for this meal.
- Opt out of the salad dressing as you already have a C and an F in the lasagna.
- Serve yourself a lot of the green salad and squeeze fresh lemon or lime over the top.
- Search for a source of protein—this meal is inadequate. If there are no additional protein options, mentally note that you will need to be on guard for additional sugar cravings before you get more protein in your body at your next meal.

The basic PFL meals help guide you to make wiser choices than you might have if you didn't have a heightened awareness. There are times to control your food down to the nitty-gritty by cooking and packing your own, and there are times like the situation I just described that you should use your PFL training to make a better decision. The chapter on Meal Construction later in this book will further educate you on the types of meals that are a part of the PFL: PVC, PVF, PVCF and PV.

This lingo for meal types is important for you to know backward and forward. As you become familiar with peak ranges for each macronutrient category, the foods that fall under each category, and the portion sizes that fit the peak range, you will free yourself from calorie counting. You will heighten your awareness of analyzing foods prepared at restaurants, family dinner parties, and recipes that have long been in your storage of favorites. This awareness is not to employ perfection, but to be empowered and make small tweaks and adjustments in order to better strategize the foods you eat.

Basic PFL Meal Structures

As you understand the blood sugar response to carbs and sugars, it is important to consider two principles of timing for having carbohydrate meals. In the basic PFL structure, I'd like you to try having your PVC meals in the first 2/3 of your waking hours and PVF meals in the final third of your day. In this way, eating strategically becomes very simple, and you adopt a strategic way of eating that is manageable and easy to remember. To repeat again, this is the *basic structure*, not the only structure.

Another highly successful structure is choosing 2-4 PVC meals (which leaves the remainder of your meals to be PVF meals) and placing them specifically around the workout—either pre- or post-workout—to optimize your body's need for energy.

Carb/Fat Combos: Red Flags!

Below are several everyday food combinations to demonstrate carbs/fat combinations you should avoid if seeking to control your body fat levels. Nearly every popular food item combines these two essential macronutrients:

- Bagel (carb) and Cream Cheese (fat)
- Pizza crust (carb) and Cheese (fat)
- Bread (carb) and Peanut Butter (fat)
- Chips (carb) and Guacamole (fat)
- Oats (carb) and Almond Butter (fat)

- Pasta (carb) and Alfredo Sauce (fat)
- Bread (carb) and Oil (fat) –popular European appetizer

"When are you going to be done following that girl's weird thing where you can't have certain foods together?" is something several of my former clients have been asked by friends or family. We laugh together as *we* understand why we do this. As we talk about the strategy, not necessity, of separating carbs and fats in meals, please don't think that foods which combine the two are bad. They're not bad, they are just not as strategic to body fat loss. By combining fats and carbs, the foods you eat become less effective and you may not reach your fat loss and fitness goals as quickly—even when watching your caloric intake. This is why you shouldn't worry intensely about calories. Concern yourself more with the combination of your power foods in proper timing intervals. If you will do this, keeping your peak ranges in mind as you select your food portions, you will give your body the variables it needs to naturally evolve to its highest-performing, healthiest state. Be sure to continue reading so you can learn more about the timing of the PVC meals, as well as when PVF meals come into play.

Conclusion

Carbs are great and most definitely not the "bad guy." If you come across any advertising that says otherwise, question the source and the agenda. Carbs simply must be used strategically to help you reach your goals. Choose complex carbs so you minimize the impact on your blood sugar, be wise about your portion sizes, and be sure to pair your carbs with a source of protein and veggies.

Carbohydrates are not the "bad guy."
Instead, they are to be respected and used wisely.

7

Fats

A re you someone who hears the word "fat" and wants to run? I used to be
this way! My fear that eating fat would *make* me fat caused me to look for
every fat-free or low-fat substitution I could find. I was horribly disillusioned
by popular belief and was an uninformed consumer. What I wish I would have
known is how to incorporate health-promoting fats into my diet without fear. I
had heard many different theories and nutrition facts on how fat was good for
me, but I couldn't understand how my body could handle more calories on top of
what I was already eating.

With the strategies of the PFL, you can put your mind at ease about
your consumption of fats as you will quickly learn the types to focus on eating. As
you implement PVF meals into your daily eating structure, you will be getting a
great serving of essential fats to optimize your brain and heart health, feel full, and
encourage fat loss.

As you learned in the previous chapter, you should focus on two
different meal combinations each day: PVC (Protein + Veggies + Carbs) and PVF
(Protein + Veggies + Fats). In our starting point basic PFL structure, replacing
your carbohydrate-based meals with fat-based meals will take place in the final
two meals of the day, whenever that is for you. Another way to think of this is in
the final third of your waking hours. Through this replacement of carbs with fats,
you will keep your blood glucose levels more stable as you prepare to sleep—the
most strategic way to promote fat loss and preserve the environment for optimal
body function.

What's So Good about the "Good" Fats

Failing to provide your body with essential fats is like sitting in a plane without a pilot and expecting the plane to take flight—there's nobody to direct the movement and make it happen. Fats have many different roles in the body that we need to appreciate and respect. Like carbohydrates, fats are used to supply energy to your body. Dietary fat is needed to absorb vitamins A, E, D, and K, all of which are very important nutrients for normal health functioning. These fat-soluble vitamins can only be absorbed when there are adequate levels of dietary fat in your system.

Without healthy fats, your body wouldn't be able to provide adequate energy, build healthy cells, or operate a healthy brain. Fats provide the structural components of cell membranes and myelin (the fatty insulating sheath that surrounds each nerve fiber) which enable the brain to carry messages faster. This means if you're incorporating healthy fats into your eating patterns, you will think more quickly and efficiently.

Fats make hormones (think of them as chemical messengers) which are extremely important in your body. Many women experience a loss of their menstrual cycle when they deprive their body of adequate fats. This can happen after a woman already has her cycle, or before a teenage girl is to begin her cycle, delaying this pubertal development.

Side note: after I learned this nutritional fact, I reflected back on my life as a teenage dancer who was very busy. My family ate very healthily and I was a lean, fit teenager. However, upon this reflection, I also recalled that good fats that I help people incorporate into their diets weren't so much on my regular list of foods at that time—I rarely ate raw nuts, avocado, coconut, or olive oil. I occasionally ate olives and cheese, but hindsight tells me that perhaps my late menstrual development at the age of 17 was due to a very low monounsaturated and polyunsaturated fats intake.

Using the PVC and PVF meal method, we can help to eliminate your fears that come from eating foods with higher calories like fat. As fats are the most concentrated source of energy of the three macronutrients, they have nine calories per gram, unlike four calories per gram in protein and carbs. You might know logically that fats are important, but still make a conscious effort to keep them out of your eating patterns. I understand the fear as yes, there are more calories in fat-based foods (even if they're "good" fats). As you remember that your blood sugar levels are more important than the overall caloric intake, you will get better and better at being able to manipulate your body composition and improve your health through PVF meals.

Let's now take a look at the types of fats that are in the foods you eat. Just as carbs are not all created equally, fats also are not all created equally.

Most of the fats and oils in the foods you eat are a mixture of saturated, monounsaturated, and polyunsaturated fats. These names are simply referring to the chemical structure of fatty acid chains. The different types of bonds that connect hydrogen to carbon atoms are what give these fats their different characteristics and effects on your body. What I hope you get from this chapter is that there are definite fats to avoid, and definite fats to make an active effort to incorporate into your food intake.

1. Trans fats are most responsible for high cholesterol. They're linked to heart disease by lowering your good cholesterol (HDL) and raising your bad cholesterol (LDL). These are formed when hydrogen is added to vegetable oil during food processing to help it solidify. This is known as hydrogenation, and is a completely foreign fat your body does not like.

Trans fats are in many candy bars, cookies, baked goods, and fast foods. Your food has Trans fats if you find any of the following phrases in the ingredient list:
    i. Hydrogenated vegetable oil
    ii. Partially hydrogenated vegetable oil
    iii. Canola Oil
    iv. Soybean Oil
    v. Rapeseed Oil
    vi. Vegetable shortening
    vii. Margarine

Trans fats may also be created if you fry a lot of your own food using vegetable oil at a high temperature.

2. Saturated fat is found in animal proteins like beef, pork, and dairy products and is the type of fat that has also been linked to the risk of heart disease. However, many recent studies are uncovering flawed data from previous studies, and are showing that saturated fats aren't necessarily the bad guy either. It's important for you to be aware of what is in your foods, and seek to eat more unsaturated fats in proportion to saturated fats. Several health-promoting fats (like coconut oil) are actually very high in saturated fat, so it's best not to play a game of black-or-white, but rather to focus on finding the balance of healthful eating using the power foods list of foods.

Foods with heart-healthy fats will still contain some saturated fats. You can't, and shouldn't, completely eliminate this fat from your diet entirely. Following the PFL recommendations will help keep your saturated fat intake to a minimum and in balance for optimal health functioning.

3. Monounsaturated fats are found in nuts, natural peanut butter, 100% extra virgin olive oil, and avocado which are specific to the PFL power fats. This type of fat can contribute to lowering your LDL (bad cholesterol) and help contribute to more vitamin E in your diet. Studies find that most Americans are deficient in this antioxidant so extra efforts here will give you positive effects in other areas.

4. Polyunsaturated fats are very good for your heart health, though these two types of fats must be balanced for optimal health function. The most recent studies on this balance indicate a 1:1 ratio of 6s to 3s is ideal:

a. Omega-6 polyunsaturated fats provide your body with essential fatty acid that your body needs but can't make on its own. These fats come from salad dressings, nuts and seeds, fast foods, cakes and pastries, pork, dairy, eggs, and beef.

b. Omega-3 polyunsaturated fats also can't be made on their own, but must come from the foods you eat. These types of fat are integral for hormones that regulate blood clotting, arterial walls control, and inflammation. These types of fat come from; fish (EPA and DHA—eicosapentaenoic acid and docosahexaenoic acid), and nuts, flaxseed, and grass-fed animal fat contributes ALA, or alpha-linolenic acid. This type of fat is often supplemented in pill form, be sure to purchase a pharmaceutical grade if you use non-food methods of getting your Omega-3s.

Foods with Essential Fats

The PFL will help you identify and utilize foods which will promote a good balance of health-promoting fats. Fats are nothing to be feared; rather, they are to be appreciated and utilized in strategic ways. Below is a list of the power fat sources that should regularly make up your PVF meals:

- Almond/Coconut/Rice Milk
- Almonds
- Almond Butter
- Almond Flour
- Avocados
- Avocado Oil
- Bacon
- Brazil Nuts

- Butter
- Cashews
- Cheese
- Chestnuts
- Chia Seeds
- Coconut
- Cream Cheese
- Egg Yolks

- Flax Seeds
- Hummus
- Macadamia Oil
- Olive Oil (100% extra virgin)
- Peanuts

- Peanut Butter
- Pecans
- Pumpkin Seeds
- Olives
- Walnuts

There may be additional foods that can fulfill the requirements to serve as a source of essential fats. After identifying the types of fats in the food you're eating, use the following loose guidelines to identify for yourself whether or not a food meets the criteria to use on a macronutrient level for a PVF meal:

- Carbs: <5 grams
- Fats: 8-12 grams*
- Calories: <200

*primarily from monounsaturated and polyunsaturated fats, though some saturated fats (like bacon) can be health-promoting when eaten 1-3 times per week.

Incorporating Fats into the PFL

Toward the end of your day—typically evening for most people's body clocks and schedules—is when you might feel especially "munchy" and want to snack on foods that could steer you away from optimal health and a body composition that gives you confidence. As you utilize your PVF meals, you should feel more satisfied than when you eat PVC meals. This is because the role of fat is different than the role of carbs and they will register different feelings in your body as you pay attention.

Fats stimulate the release of CCK (Cholecystokinin), a hormone which sends a signal to your brain that you've eaten enough food to be satisfied. Fats also slow down the digestion of the food you've eaten so your blood sugar levels stay more stable. In the previous chapter on carbohydrates, you learned that it's ideal to keep your blood sugar as stable as possible to promote fat loss. When your blood sugar doesn't significantly rise, it can't significantly fall—this prevents cravings from hitting when you're working so hard to reach your goals.

Fake Butter?!

Fats that shouldn't have any place in your kitchen or your stomach include "fake" butters like *I Can't Believe It's Not Butter!*, *Smart Balance*, or *Betty Crocker*

Spreads (there are many more!). Anything that has been processed and manufactured in a factory to reach a lower, more appealing caloric and macronutrient number may actually harm your body more than help it. These processed, butter-like substances are full of artificial ingredients, artificial colors, and synthetic vitamins that do nothing to boost your immune system. The process by which these spreads are made is called "interesterification," which has been thought by many food scientists to be more dangerous to your health than Trans fats.

Let's move on to fake butters' cousin, margarine. This butter-like product is very high in Trans-fatty acids, contributes to higher cholesterol, and decreases your body's response to insulin. Butter, on the other hand, is rich in fat-soluble vitamins A, E, and K, and is a healthier source of saturated fats. When used in balance with other power fats, butter is a great source of completing a PVF meal and keeping your energy intake balanced for fat loss.

Keep in mind that the strategy of separating your carbs and fats may keep you from eating foods you're used to—like bread and butter. You will quickly learn that you really don't need to butter your toast. The grain is very delicious on its own, or even better to use a different carbohydrate source in the morning. At the end of the day, remember that I'm teaching you principles of which to be aware, not to make you miserable. Use them however you see fit to best improve your health and manipulate your body composition.

Clean Up your Baked Goods Recipes

In nearly all baking recipes, a very simple and delicious substitute you can use for butter or margarine is unsweetened applesauce. Not only is it much better for your health and waistline, but it makes your foods extra moist. Try this substitution in your brownies, cookies, and cakes. Keeping unsweetened applesauce as a regularly-stocked item in your pantry is an excellent way to lighten up the foods and desserts you love and utilize at your indulgence meals. You will find that I use unsweetened applesauce in many of the baked goods recipes in the Power Foods Lifestyle Recipe Books, available on www.body-buddies.com.

Plain Greek yogurt can also serve as a nutritional super-star for substitution. This simple swap can increase the protein in your meal and significantly decrease the non-strategic fats and sugars in the food you eat. Try substituting Greek yogurt for:

- Mayonnaise in salad dressings
- Mayonnaise in deviled eggs
- Cream cheese in cheesecake recipes

- Cream in cream-based sauces like alfredo sauce
- Syrup on top of waffles and pancakes
- Butter on sides like potatoes
- Sour cream in Mexican dishes
- Milk in smoothies
- Mayonnaise in tuna mixtures
- Also try marinating meat and seafood in Greek yogurt instead of oil

What about Egg Yolks?

Egg yolks are a great source of saturated and monunsaturated fats while contributing dietary cholesterol. Unfortunately, this cholesterol awareness is what causes many people to steer away from eating yolks. This is due to the 1990s and the mass media that was current at the time—it has since been refuted and dietary cholesterol has found to contribute only slightly to elevated blood cholesterol. Our previous discussion on Trans fats is what you should remember most—those are the greatest contributor to elevated blood cholesterol.

Instead of fearing the egg yolk, respect it. It is a power fat with approximately 4.5 grams per yolk. This means that to fulfill a peak range of power fat for a PVF meal, you should eat 2 yolks, or 1 yolk and get another 3.5-7.5 grams of fat from an additional power fat like avocado or coconut oil. If you choose to eat a full egg for breakfast, keep in mind that you should limit the carbs that are in that meal. Continue to remember that the PFL principles are two-fold: promoting optimal internal health function while providing manipulation of energy nutrients to achieve an aesthetic appeal externally. It's possible to achieve both goals when you think and eat strategically.

Thoughts on Oils

There are a few reasons to replace the oils you may have regularly stocked in your pantry with those listed on the power fats list.

1. Canola oil is manufactured at high temperatures using a mechanical process that involves toxic chemicals. These high temperatures can change the omega-3 content of the oil, destroy vitamin E, and significantly raise the oil's Trans-fatty acids and saturated fats.

2. Vegetable oils are manufactured in a factory, usually from genetically modified (GMO) crops that have been heavily treated with pesticides.

A GMO crop is one where the DNA has been modified using genetic engineering techniques. GMOs have been linked to many diseases, including gastrointestinal and immune system disorders, accelerated aging, and infertility. It is best to keep these out of your body.

3. Vegetable oils contain a very high number of polyunsaturated fats, instead of a more stable ratio of polyunsaturated to monounsaturated fats. Your body needs fats for rebuilding cells and hormone production, but it has to use the building blocks you give it. If you take in a high concentration of polyunsaturated fats instead of proper ratios, your body will naturally use these fats in building and creating new cells—in other words, put on fat.

4. Partially hydrogenated soybean oil contains Trans fat. *Check your labels—you might choke when you see just how many of your everyday foods and snacks contain this silent thief of your health.* In addition to that, most corn and soy crops are genetically engineered, the DNA modification of which has been thought to put human health at risk.

In using 100% extra virgin olive oil, be aware of how to find the real deal. A study by the University of California in 2008 found that as much as 69% of imported European olive oil sold as extra virgin in grocery stores was not actually virgin olive oil. In most cases, extra virgin olive oil is mixed with a lower grade olive oil, and not even from the same country. Sometimes, even vegetable or canola oil is used. The resulting blend is then chemically changed so it can't be discovered and sold as extra virgin to the manufacturing company. To ensure you're getting the best olive oil for your health, be sure to do these two things:

1. Check the label of your oil and be sure it is labeled "Extra Virgin"—not "pure," "light," or "olive oil." These categories of oil have gone through chemical refinement.

2. Check the label for the country or vineyard from which the olive has come—if there are multiple countries listed, the process listed above certainly was used.

Conclusion

Rather than fearing the calories in fat, learn to balance the power fats you eat in PVF meals. You now know how to use your essential fats strategically. Keep your serving size for each fat-based food in PVF meals between 8-12 grams (as a starting point for most healthy adults), and only eat that high of a healthy fat serving in the absence of a power carbohydrate source. If you focus on a higher carb intake, consider decreasing the portion size of your fat source. A healthy intake of fats will contribute to a healthier and fitter body.

Fats are essential for our bodies.
Learning to eat them strategically is the best way to ensure
your success in health and aesthetics.

8

Vegetables

When I was a young girl, I allegedly told my mom that I wanted to be just like her—I wanted to grow up to "watch Perry Mason and eat peas on my salad!" I was fortunate to have parents who taught me by example that vegetables are an integral part of daily nutritional habits.

You most likely know how important vegetables are to your health; yet even while knowing this, perhaps you still have a hard time eating them. There are a few understandable reasons for this:

1. They can be expensive.
2. They don't stay fresh for long.
3. They have odd textures.
4. They take too long to prepare.
5. They can taste disgusting if not prepared right.
6. You may have an allergy (yes, some people do!)

If you're someone who has a hard time getting your vegetables down (let's call 'em veggies from here on out), you might find new motivation through my explanations about why they are an essential part of your daily eating habits. One of the easiest changes you can make to improve your health is simply by including more vegetables in what you eat every day.

As I go about my day-to-day activities, I often find myself in conversations centered on nutrition with anyone and everyone. Whether it's the bank teller, grocery store cashier, postal worker, or crossing guard, I ultimately try to leave every person with a touch of the PFL—the challenge to drink more water and have a serving of vegetables with every meal. Those are the starting points for anybody trying be just a little bit better and feel a little more vibrant each day.

Have you ever felt super downtrodden, fatigued, and that your brain isn't functioning at its best? This could very well be due to low veggie intake. The main job of veggies is to provide fiber, vitamins, and minerals to your body, thereby facilitating metabolic reactions that release energy. They amplify the way you feel as you're eating balanced meals with your foods in PVC and PVF combinations. This is why you will experience so much more energy when you replace processed foods with foods from the power foods list; you're "unlocking" your body's ability to utilize the nutrients in your food.

For the purposes of the PFL, let's consider veggies to be a separate category than the macronutrients of power protein, carbs, and fats. Though veggies are technically classified as a complex carbohydrate due to their high fiber content, we will keep them in their own "family."

Just How Many Vegetables Should I Eat?

Following the PFL means including a serving of vegetables at every meal. The use of the capital 'V' in PVC and PVF meals means 1-2 cups—about the size of your fist or so. Following this recommendation will put you around 6–12 cups of vegetables daily, which is very much in line with the Center for Disease Control and Prevention's recommendation. You can calculate your body's specific needs on their website and adjust your intake accordingly.[6]

Think of how much more energy you will feel by fueling your body with vital nutrients every 2.5–3 hours (which you will learn more about in the Meal Timing chapter). The changes you may experience over both the short and long-term are incredible, including helping to manage, prevent, and even sometimes reverse chronic disease, injury, and illness. I've seen many miracles in the past few years of working with people, and I am grateful for the power of nutrition in giving each of us a higher quality of life. Now, if only we will apply this knowledge!

Take your time—if you've hardly eaten veggies, you might want to work your way up to eating six servings per day. If you jump right in, your digestive tract might have a rough adjustment. Dramatic increases in fiber may cause a small amount of bloating and/or gas. If this happens, be patient and persistent. Your body will soon adapt and begin processing as it should with a plethora of nutrients in your system that will work over the course of time to aid your body.

---

[6] http://www.cdc.gov/nutrition/everyone/fruitsvegetables/

As I mentioned previously, try to eat one serving of vegetables every time you eat a meal. Yes, even at breakfast, otherwise known as Meal 1. Doing so will help you feel full throughout the day and keep you more regular thanks to the fiber content. (If you are wanting to juice your veggies, that's fine. You'll get the vitamins and minerals, but you remove the fibrous content, so be aware of that and seek to get some of your veggies in their natural form). Toward the end of the day as you are finding yourself dealing with the desire to eat more, you might consider allowing yourself veggies in greater quantity. I encourage you not to think of foods as unlimited (as every food you put in your body will have a reaction in your body), but as having a good go-to option if you're feeling the urge to eat. Obviously eating more veggies instead of brownies and ice cream is a better option. Try to keep your end-of-day veggies limited to leafy greens as much as possible, though if you really want carrots, green beans, or a bell pepper—for heaven's sakes, don't resist. Along with the strategy of the PVF meal combination, additional leafy greens will help you fight the desire to eat sugary, high-fat foods.

Don't Be One of Them

I find it very interesting that every time a new study comes out and is publicized, many people tend to go a bit overboard in their implementation of the research. It makes me roll my eyes when I hear individuals talking about how they've read a new study, so now they're "going to eat a certain food 3x daily for its benefits."

Tomatoes have been proven to help reduce the risk of cancer!
Cauliflower has many antioxidants that help protect you from free-radical damage!

Broccoli has been proven to reduce blood cholesterol and prevent Type 2 Diabetes!

Oh, really? Tell me more! How intriguing!

They're vegetables—*of course* they have great health benefits. Why have we been taught to eat them from the time we were children? Let me let you in on a little secret:

All vegetables help prevent and reduce the risk of disease...

...the key is to include a good variety of vegetables regularly. When a new study comes out and is plastered all over the TV, magazines, and social media, don't go ballistic and stock up your fridge and pantry with only that particular vegetable (this principle is true for any food group—not just vegetables). Instead, give your body the best possible health benefits by constantly exposing yourself to a variety of veggies.

Here's what I suggest: Choose 4-5 varieties of vegetable each week as you grocery shop. The following week, you can change it up and shift to a few new varieties. Don't overstock your fridge crisper with veggies as this may cause them to go bad before you're able to use them. I find that the "4-5-variety" rule helps you to have a moderate change-up for the week and not get bored with your veggies without letting the produce go bad.

Why You Need Vegetables

1. Vegetables are high in vitamins and minerals. Vitamins work synergistically to promote proper muscle contraction, as well as to help prevent muscle spasms.

2. Vegetables are low in calories, which is great news for anyone attempting to lower their daily caloric intake and lose body fat. Even though we don't actively count calories while following the PFL, they do matter. Keeping calories lower than your body's maintenance level is an important element to consider along with pairing your macros wisely when planning meals.

3. Vegetables are high in fiber. Consuming fiber not only helps you feel full and keep your body digestion "regular," but also normalizes your blood sugar levels to reduce hormonally-triggered food cravings. Power-housing your way through insatiable cravings can become quite difficult and overwhelming. Wouldn't you want to reduce the number of cravings by increasing your dietary fiber intake through vegetable consumption?

4. Vegetables repair damaged DNA. More specifically, cruciferous vegetables have been linked to decreased risk for several types of cancers including lung, prostate, breast, and colon cancer. Among the most well-known cruciferous vegetables are broccoli, broccoli sprouts, and cabbage. In other words, eating vegetables gives your body the tools it needs to prevent disease. In our current society, this should be a huge motivating factor.

5. Vegetables prevent age-associated mental decline. This becomes more important as you begin to age and realize how quickly your thought processes and memories begin to dull.

Natural vs. Artificial Nutrients

So why can't you just take a vitamin? It's easier, faster, and doesn't have a taste and texture that many people find repulsive. While supplementing your meals with vitamins may make it easier to get your nutrients and minimize food preparation time, your body's absorption rate increases and operates more efficiently when you get your vitamins by consuming real food.

Study after study shows that, when taken in pill form, only a fraction of the vitamin amounts listed on the label of the bottle are actually absorbed into your body. In other words, you're basically wasting your money by not getting the full dose of the vitamins you think you are. Eating vegetables and getting your nutrients through real food amplifies the absorption of vitamins and minerals in your system, including many that would otherwise be eliminated by the body if taken only in pill form.

If you use a superfood complex or any variety of powders designed to give you the vitamins and minerals in veggies, I still encourage you to aim for at least four of your six servings of veggies in whole form at every meal.

Below is a very basic list of popular vegetables, and a great place to start if you're someone who has rarely integrated vegetables into your lifestyle. There most definitely are other vegetables out there that are packed with nutrients and health benefits; this list simply represents some basics. Feel free to venture outside of these options:

- Arugula
- Asparagus
- Bell Pepper
- Broccoli
- Brussels sprouts
- Carrots
- Cauliflower
- Celery
- Collard Greens
- Cucumber
- Edamame
- Egg Plant
- Green Beans
- Jicama
- Kale
- Mushrooms
- Mustard Greens
- Romaine Lettuce
- Spaghetti Squash
- Spinach
- Summer Squash
- Sweet Peppers
- Tomatoes
- Zucchini

Methods of Preparation

When adapting to your new lifestyle, the food you eat should be as close as possible to real, meaning you should avoid canned and processed vegetables whenever possible. Shopping several times a week for fresh produce is definitely worth it in terms of what is best for your body! Even frozen vegetables are better than canned, and nearly as good as fresh. Time is a factor for many people, and I whole-heartedly agree with the phrase, "At least it's better than not eating them." With that said, find what works best for your lifestyle; if that means doing the best you can with canned and frozen vegetables, that is just fine.

If you dread eating vegetables, know that it doesn't need to be that way. The taste and texture of produce is dependent upon your method of preparation. Be creative and experiment with new ways of cooking to find preparation techniques that work for you. When you find what you like, you'll eat it! Be sure to give the recipes in the Power Foods Lifestyle Recipe Books a try!

As you figure out what works for you, keep in mind that light, heat, air, acid, and cooking fluids can damage the vitamins in your vegetables. The more you do to maximize the taste of your vegetables by altering them from their raw form, the more you destroy their nutrients and they become an "empty calorie food." Try to minimize their exposure to heat, air, and cooking water. Raw vegetables can actually increase the rate of your metabolism as it takes more energy to break them down and digest them. However, maybe you don't like the taste of raw veggies, or have an allergy where you can't eat them raw (yes, it exists and affects many). For these populations, steaming via stovetop or microwaving can often be the best cooking methods to use. These methods use a small amount of water and provide limited exposure to heat. Is this to say that any other form of preparation (boiling, baking, etc.) is no good? Not at all. Remember that everything we discuss in the PFL is to increase your awareness so you can make the best choices for you and your lifestyle.

Be sure to wash your veggies before preparing them or eating them raw. If you struggle with the flavor of vegetables, adding a little seasoned salt (no MSG), garlic salt, oregano, Italian seasoning, celery salt, or spicy brown mustard can add some zesty flavor and makes eating them a much more enjoyable experience.

Do I Have to Buy Organic?

At the end of the day, we all have a budget to which we must align our grocery purchases. You may or may not be able to afford organic produce. People frequently approach me with skepticism about this trend in eating. Is organic produce just hype, a fad that will pass in coming years? Is this method of eating for an elitist class?

The short answer is 'no'. The reality of the modern agricultural industry is that fruits and vegetables are sprayed with pesticides and coated in chemical residue. We must grapple with the balance between purchasing affordable produce and eating foods that aren't grown and treated using harmful chemicals. The government sets "safe" pesticide residue limits on produce, and your local grocery store must abide by these rules. However, many groups outside the government argue that any chemical interference with food is harmful and do their best to inform the public of the most dangerous, chemically-modified foods available for purchase. These foods, they argue, should be purchased organically.

One of these groups is called The Environmental Working Group. Each year, this group analyzes data from the Department of Agriculture[7] and puts out an annual list of their findings. Entitled "The Dirty Dozen," the research compiled by the Environmental Working Group compares the amount of pesticide residue on foods and ranks them according to how much or little they have. This organization says that buying the dirty dozen organically, rather than traditionally, will reduce the exposure to pesticides by 80%.

I hope you will use this information to decide for yourself whether you feel the need to purchase your produce organically or not. I believe in a hierarchy of eating, which means you progress from principle to principle without turning into a black-or-white, all-or-nothing person. If you are already eating a balanced and PFL-friendly way, then perhaps you are at a point where you might heavily consider purchasing more organic and non-GMO foods. However, if you are at a point where you're going to start cooking at home for the first time and stop using burgers, fries, and pizza as meals, then perhaps you can work up to eating organically. Be careful not to jump to a higher principle of health before you have mastered the basics. This applies to every aspect of the PFL. There is a great degree of learning, application, and mastery to fully live the PFL to the level that best suits you and what you'd like to accomplish both with your internal health and external appearance.

Conclusion

Increasing the amount of vegetables you eat each day will go a long way to help you accomplish both your short-term and long-term health and body composition goals. The increase in vitamins, minerals, and fiber will help your body to function efficiently with maximum energy. Be sure to try new vegetables constantly, taking joy in the great variety of colors, textures, tastes, and vitamins provided by your local grocery store or Farmers' market.

---

[7] Environmental Working Group. http://www.ewg.org/foodnews/summary.php

9

Fruits

Fruit is delicious, easy to eat on the go, and a wonderful contributor to your everyday health. When you eat a variety of fruit, you are nourished with vitamins, minerals, antioxidants, fiber, and phytochemicals. For many years, the government's food pyramid has taught us that several pieces of fruit per day are part of a healthy lifestyle. Yes, this is true, fruit is part of a healthy lifestyle.

However, America's population is growing more and more obese each year. When you fall into the category of needing to lose a significant number (20+ pounds) of body fat, you need to act now. You may already be experiencing the impacts of higher-than-average body fat on your quality of life. When you are uncomfortable and needing a change, I encourage you to utilize every possible strategy to make the change in the most efficient way possible. One of these strategies is eliminating most fruits from your eating method *for the duration of your fat loss efforts.*

I whole-heartedly believe fruit should be a part of your regular food intake. However, there are many controversial studies out there that state both you should, or shouldn't, eat fruit while working to eliminate body fat. Remember what this entire book is about: learning principles of nutritional science to implement in your lifestyle. You must learn a principle and then make a decision about whether you feel that is a principle worth applying in your health efforts at the present moment. In this chapter, I would like to outline a few characteristics of fruit that may be sabotaging your fat loss efforts, and leave it to you to decide what is best in your personal situation.

As fruit is associated with the term "healthy," all too many people believe that eating fruit will help them lose weight. While arguably true, that "weight loss" can actually be a very detailed and complicated issue. If eating fruit is causing you to eat less of the normal foods you regularly eat, resulting in a greater caloric deficit, then yes, this will help you lose weight if you are 15+ pounds overweight. I have found, however, that those who are so close to a more defined and chiseled physique are preventing the results they want to see by eating the wrong types of fruit and eating them at the wrong times.

My goal behind this discussion on fruit is to keep in mind the role of insulin in fat loss—this is the underlying success of the PFL methodology. The principles of food combinations, portions, and timing are to help keep your blood sugar from either dropping or rising too drastically. The more you stabilize your blood sugar levels, the more you are burning fat, increasing your energy, and putting your body in a nutrient-absorbing environment. This environment has helped so many people who follow the PFL to reverse many health conditions, including pre-diabetes, insulin resistance, and indicators of metabolic syndrome: high triglycerides, high blood pressure, and high cholesterol. Absorbing micronutrients and helping your body eliminate fat stores are both critical to your body functioning at its best.

But Fructose is a Natural Sugar!

Let's look at fructose, the natural sugar in fruit. While fructose and glucose are both monosaccharaides (simple-unit sugars), they are processed differently in your body and have diverse metabolic effects.

Glucose bypasses the liver for removal where fructose does not. Through a complicated process called fructolysis, fructose goes through some chemical changes in the liver. Only after this process does it resemble glucose, your body's primary source of energy. These newly-structured molecules now can enter the pathways that glucose takes to produce energy.

Many studies have found that fructose does not raise blood sugar levels as dramatically as glucose; however, it's critical to note the other side of the coin. The price for this possible benefit is the liver rapidly up taking the fructose and converting it into triglycerides. This is something you want to avoid as it elevates your risk for a stroke.

Diets high in fructose have been linked to higher rates of metabolic syndrome in studies with rats. Additional studies[8] have shown that a high-fructose diet increases visceral body fat due to insulin resistance, a state where your body is not as responsive to insulin, which tells your cells to absorb active energy. In the typical American diet, higher fructose intake is not actually coming from fruits, but from high fructose corn syrup in soda, fruit drinks, cookies, and cereal. The PFL will help you not only eliminate those very non-strategic foods, but use fruit in a more efficient way.

---

[8] http://www.ncbi.nlm.nih.gov/pmc/articles/PMC2682989/

The PFL Recommendation

I personally stick to only a few fruits on a regular basis, and utilize the others in my indulgence meals or enjoy as a special carbohydrate exchange. The fruits I regularly consume and recommend for you as well include blueberries, raspberries, strawberries, grapefruit, bananas, oranges, and apples.

When you look at fruit with a strategic fat loss mindset, you need to look at their glycemic load. The simple explanation of glycemic load is a food's ability to break down (quickly or slowly) and how that breakdown influences blood sugar. As you should try to keep blood sugar levels as stable as possible, gravitate toward the foods that are lower in glycemic load. The fruits I named above all happen to be lower on the glycemic index. Their properties are such that they don't impact your blood sugar levels as much as other fruits (of course, given the right portion, they possibly could. We are talking about a ½ cup of fruit here).

Even when eating lower glycemic-load fruits, you should be strategic about *when* you eat them. Fruit should ideally come either in your pre- or post-workout meals (assuming your workout isn't at the end of the day). This is when your body can better handle the increase in sugar (fructose in fruit) more efficiently. Your body will also capitalize on this timing because your raised blood sugar will facilitate better absorption of the protein from your meal. Does this mean you should never eat fruit at nighttime? Isn't it a carb, and you want to keep carbs out of pre-bedtime meals? Not necessarily. Sometimes having a fruit with a protein and vegetable gives you that little bit of "sweet" you need at the end of a long day, and can be more beneficial in the long run. This might help keep you consistently following this lifestyle rather than taking the all-or-nothing approach, and crashing and burning like every other diet out there. What matters most here is that you remember when it's most strategic to place fruit, then let your daily psychological and emotional state be your barometer for deciding just how much to "dial it in."

One of the yummiest evening meals I will eat is ½ c. cottage cheese (2%) with 4 large strawberries and ½ cucumber. That's technically a PVc meal, but if it keeps me away from the brownies and ice cream, golly whiz, let's go for that PVc. Are you catching my drift? Progress, not perfection, is our goal. There is a time and a place to comply strictly to these principles if you wish to achieve your physique's optimal shape and aesthetic look. As I train competitors and compete myself, there are phases of weeks where we simply practice higher discipline and dial in with more of a "diet mentality," then scale back to our lifestyle mentality at the conclusion of the competition. That is how we avoid the rebound trap into which many others fall. The PFL is our baseline way of functioning—a true lifestyle, not a diet.

Dried Fruit?

"Is dried fruit something I can eat?" many people ask. You also may have heard that dried fruit is healthy because, well, it's fruit! So that's good, right?

Of course you can eat it—you can eat whatever you would like, duh (catch my lovely sarcasm here with a wink). Instead, your question should be, "will dried fruit contribute to my goal of losing body fat?" You might substitute any food in the place for "dried fruit" and get in the habit of using this question, rather than using definitive words such as "good" and "bad," or "I can't eat that" versus "I can eat that."

In answer to the question, my answer is a rigid 'no.' Dried fruit is far too high in carbohydrates and sugar to help blood sugar levels stay in check and keep metabolism revved.

"But, Kristy," I can hear you saying. "You said this book is about a healthy lifestyle. I don't want to cut fruit out of my eating habits forever. How long should I stick to this method?"

That's a great question and one you should be asking. Cut the majority of fruit out of your eating habits, and focus on strategic use of it instead, for as long as you are working to lose body fat. This may be for a few weeks or months, depending on how consistently you follow this method of eating. If you stick to the PFL very closely, you should be able to reach your goals at a quick, yet healthy rate (0.5–3 pounds per week), find that happiness and contentment for which you have been looking, and then begin maintenance mode. Maintenance mode is where you allow an increase in portion size of each macronutrient category per meal, while still keeping the integrity of the meal. You might also have an extra indulgence meal in maintenance mode. I'll cover this more in a later chapter.

Whether you are in the fat loss portion of the PFL, maintenance mode, or muscle growth mode, fruit counts as a serving of carbohydrates (even if it is not a fruit that is on the power foods list.) This means that when you eat a fruit—let's take an apricot for example—it should be combined with a source of protein and vegetables. Turn that plain apricot into a small dessert by dicing it into a serving of cottage cheese and eating some celery on the side. Voila! A Power Foods Meal.

What about Fruit Juice?

Let's first keep in mind that fructose, the natural sugar in fruit, is not processed in your body the same as glucose, so just because it's natural doesn't always mean it's beneficial for health and body composition changes.

The following are a few interesting facts that you should know about the Food and Drug Administration (FDA) and their rules9 concerning product labels:

1. If a beverage claims that it contains fruit or vegetable juice, you will also find the percentage of juice on the information label near the top. If a food label does not claim to contain fruit or vegetable juice, it may still have photos of fruits and vegetables and not be breaking any rules. This can cause you to falsely assume the beverage has real juice.

2. When a beverage uses a small percentage of real juice, it is okay if they describe the product as "flavored," but you will not see the word "juice" listed in the ingredient list.

3. Beverages that are 100% juice may be called "juice" but beverages that are diluted to less than 100% must have the word "juice" qualified with a term like "beverage," "drink," or "cocktail." It may also have the word "diluted" with the name of the juice following.

4. Juices made from concentrate must be labeled with that term or "reconstituted" which will be a part of the name as it appears on the label. This labeling can be no smaller than ½ the size of the name of the juice. This rule is only effective for beverages that claim it's a specific juice. That means "fruit punch" and "lemonade," because they do not include the name of a specific juice, do not need to use the terms "from concentrate" or "reconstituted."

5. There is no rule that keeps companies from using photos of fruits and vegetables that are not proportionate to the percentage of juice the beverage actually contains.

I hope this opens your eyes into just how deceptive beverages can be. Use your new knowledge to start looking more closely at food labels and becoming your own personal chief inspector of the foods you choose to eat. Your personal responsibility and desire to increase awareness will make the biggest difference as new foods continue to be placed on grocery and convenience store shelves.

Conclusion

Fruit is wonderful and healthy! It gives you much nourishment that your body needs to help prevent and fight illness and disease. Keeping this in mind, the way you

---

[9] http://www.fda.gov/Food/GuidanceRegulation/GuidanceDocumentsRegulatoryInformation/LabelingNutrition/ucm064872.htm

strategically use fruits in your eating style will have an impact on the outcome of your efforts. A good strategy is one that helps you reach your goals and maintain them efficiently.

Utilizing strategies in all that you do helps to eliminate the pervasive negative cycle of feeling like a failure, although you are putting forth great effort. Let your efforts to gain control of your life and your health work in favor for you. This is why it would be wise for you to try eating fruit strategically and remember that fruit should be eaten in moderation.

10
Meal Construction

W hen you mail a letter to someone, do you simply put the paper in the mail? I highly doubt that—it would get nowhere fast. We are trained from the time we are young to package a piece of mail correctly by putting the contents in an envelope, sealing it shut, completing the return and recipient addresses, then stamping the envelope. This allows the contents to pass through the postal system. We don't think twice about this process, do we?

Eating a meal is very similar to this process. My guess is that you haven't been trained to package your meals correctly in a way that keeps your metabolism functioning at a high rate, your blood sugar levels stabilized, and your body absorbing maximum vitamins and minerals. Just as you need to complete all parts of preparing a letter for sending, you need to make sure all components of a proper meal are in place if you wish for it to be effectively utilized in your body. No longer should you think in terms of caloric values, but think in terms of complete meals in appropriate portion sizes. This is what we call the *integrity of a meal*—proper macronutrient categories being present.

Choosing to follow the PFL principles may initially appear that you are depriving yourself of many foods. While it may be easy to feel this way while eating healthy foods the majority of the time, you are actually giving your body the greatest gift! You will realize just how much food is a blessing. It truly is when you remember that many people don't have access to nutritious foods to fuel their bodies.

Let's review the representation of macronutrient categories:

$$P = Protein$$
$$C = Carbohydrate$$

$$F = Fat$$
$$V = Veggie$$

An upper-case letter indicates a full peak range of that particular category of foods. Therefore, the peak ranges for capital letters are as follows:

P = Protein (15-30 g)
C = Carbohydrate (20-30 g)
F = Fat (8-12 g)
V = Veggie (1 -2 c.)

What about lower-case letters? You may see myself or a Body Buddies coach use this representation when describing a meal and wonder what it means. The lower-case letter indicates a half peak range portion size (or enough to be significant, but still falling short of a full peak range), where a double upper-case letter indicates a double peak range portion size.

p = Protein (7.5-15 g)
c = Carbohydrate (10-15 g)
f = Fat (4-6 g)
v = Veggie (1/2-1 c.)

PP = Protein (30-60 g)
CC = Carbohydrate (40-60 g)
FF= Fat (16-24 g)
VV= Veggie (2-4 c.–no need to be excessive here)

Basic Structure of the Power Foods Lifestyle

Meal 1	P + V + C
Meal 2	P + V + C
Meal 3	P + V + C
Meal 4	P + V + C
Meal 5	P + V + F
Meal 6	P + V + F

As you can see, protein is consistently a part of every meal. Veggies also appear in every meal. But fats and carbs are separated and used strategically at different times of the day.

Is this to say you can't have a power fat earlier in the day? No, not at all. Is this to say you can't have a power carb before bed? No, not at all. I'll get into additional structures of the PFL you may utilize at the end of this chapter. However, I encourage you to eat according to this structure first for a few weeks, and from there, branch out to finding a variation of PVC and PVF meals that works best for you. This is because the average American is eating a heavy carbohydrate diet. Cutting these too quickly can produce quick results initially but may cause your body to plateau. We want to instead work our way down into only using enough carbs for your body's needs. This could be anywhere from 0-5 PVC meals each day.

Use the basic PFL structure above as your "home base" to return to if you are not satisfied with your results—it will be a strong foundation that will get you back to a structured and maintainable approach. The key is to make PVC and PVF meals your typical way of eating—that is why we call it a lifestyle.

Convert Macros to Real Food

This is the part of meal planning that I really enjoy—application of the scientific principles we have talked about so far. Selecting the foods that will form your meals all begins with looking at your power foods chart (be sure to refer to the last page of the book for your quick-reference chart you can use when planning and shopping).

For the basic PFL structure, all of your PVC meals (meals 1–4) should fall in the first 2/3 of your waking hours and your PFV meals (meals 5-6) should come in the final 1/3 of your waking hours. The timing of your meals is relative to your schedule and body clock. Be sure to read the Meal Timing chapter thoroughly to plan your meal times for your individual schedule.

Below are three examples of basic meal plans. The most important parts of putting together your meal plan for the day (or I recommend you do it on a weekly basis), is to identify the foods and portions first, and then get creative with how you will combine those foods into a delicious and appetizing meal. These plans are very basic, while the Power Foods Recipe Books show you more creative ways to make PVC and PVF meals.

Example Meal Plan One

Meal 1:   (P) 4 egg whites
                  (C) ½ cup oats
                  (V) 1 cup spinach

Meal 2:   (P) ½ cup cottage cheese (2%)
                  (C) ½ cup blueberries
                  (V) ½ medium cucumber

Meal 3:   (P) 4 oz. can tuna (packed in water)
                  (C) 3 oz. yam
                  (V) 1 cup broccoli

Meal 4:   (P) 1 serving protein powder
                  (C) ½ apple
                  (V) ½ bell pepper

Meal 5:   (P) 4 oz. grilled chicken breast
                  (F) 2 oz. sliced avocado
                  (V) 1 cup steamed zucchini

Meal 6:   (P) 1 serving protein powder
                  (F) 1 Tbsp. 100% natural peanut butter
                  (V) 1 cup green beans

Example Meal Plan Two

Meal 1:   (P) 4 oz. fried turkey breast
                  (C) 1 slice 100% whole wheat toast (no butter)
                  (V) ½ raw bell pepper

Meal 2:   (P) 1 serving protein powder
                  (C) 1/2 medium banana
                  (V) 1 cup spinach

Meal 3:   (P) 4 oz. lean ground turkey (99% lean)
                  (C) 3 oz. baked red potato
                  (V) 1 cup asparagus

Meal 4:   (P) 3 oz. chicken breast
              (C) 1 tortilla (100% whole wheat)
              (V) 1 Roma tomato

Meal 5:   (P) 4 oz. wild-caught tilapia
              (F) 2 tsp. 100% extra virgin olive oil
              (V) 1 cup cauliflower

Meal 6:   (P) ½ cup cottage cheese (2%)
              (F) 12 raw almonds
              (V) 2 stalks celery

Example Meal Plan Three

Meal 1:   (P) 1 serving protein powder
              (C) 1/2 orange
              (V) 1 cup kale

Meal 2:   (P) 4 oz. tofu
              (C) ½ cup black beans
              (V) 1 cup carrots

Meal 3:   (P) 4 oz. wild-caught halibut
              (C) ½ cup brown rice
              (V) 1 cup summer squash

Meal 4:   (P) 1 serving protein powder
              (C) ½ cup oats
              (V) 10 baby carrots

Meal 5:   (P) 4 oz. chicken breast
              (F) 1 Tbsp. coconut oil
              (V) 1 cup mushrooms

Meal 6:   (P) 4 hard-boiled egg whites
              (F) 10 large black olives + 1 egg yolk
              (V) 2 c. leafy mustard greens

Be Patient with Your Body

During your first few weeks of following the PFL, your body will need to adapt to eating nutrient-packed foods. At first, your body may not digest them as easily because you have allowed it to get used to eating foods that perhaps weren't as packed with nutrients. Just keep at it and trust your body will adjust. Learn to focus on the fact that you're now fueling your body and re-training every cell to function optimally, which takes time. Keep at it and focus on behavioral changes more than being hyper-focused on results.

If turning to healthy foods has been a major shift for you, stomachaches may be a slight symptom for the first few days. This is due to the high fiber content in the vegetables you will be consuming regularly. Be patient—the stomachaches will subside. If constipation occurs due to the higher protein intake, be sure that you are drinking plenty of water and try squeezing fresh lemon into your water in the morning. The lemon won't necessarily aid digestion, but many dietitians' theory is that the refreshing taste of the water will help you be sure to drink plenty of it, thus aiding in constipation relief.

As you consistently put strategic food combinations and portions in your body, the absorption and digestion process will become almost mechanical. Your body will quickly recognize the foods as if it were saying, *Hey, I know how to process this. Keep it coming!*

Other Structures of the Power Foods Lifestyle

No two bodies are created equally. In the time that has passed since the first edition of this book was published, I have worked with and seen so many bodies, disorders, and complexities. Experimenting with variations of PVC and PVF combinations has been more than eye-opening into how different populations may use the same terminology, but create a different strategy to living this lifestyle. That's just it—the PFL should give you knowledge and tools to essentially live any variation that works best for you, and be your best at living it consistently! To qualify as living a PFL what matters most is that you are doing the following:

1. Putting strategic power foods in your body the majority of the time.

2. Packaging your meals with "meal integrity" as PVC, PVF, or PVCF meals.

3. Planning and preparing your foods so that you have structure and personal accountability.

With that said, let's dive into a few other variations you might consider trying to see how it feels in your body. In the Body Buddies Podcast, I often talk about how every statement in the nutrition and fitness industry should have an asterisk at the end with the reference "exceptions always apply." With so many genetics, upbringings, allergies, and pre-dispositions to food, there must be workarounds. And there are.

With the following examples, please take into consideration that some people can and do function better on a daily total of 70-100 grams of carbohydrates. Due to this, we can get away with 2–3 PVC meals in a day and help you feel you have enough energy. What matters here is consistency and compliance in order to determine which method is truly best for you. Until you develop the mental discipline to follow through and learn how your body works best, you will continue to feel haphazard in your efforts, and that your body may be betraying you. I urge you to consider scheduling a consultation, or go through our Custom Coaching program which is personally tailored to you by one of the Body Buddies coaches. You may learn more at www.body-buddies.com. You can do this on your own but you need to be determined.

Demographic Profile: Sedentary all day but works out most days in the evening.

Recommendation: Package the PVC meals around the workout—2 prior to and 1 post workout.

Warning: Make your carbs that are close to bedtime are those lower on the glycemic index to keep your blood sugar levels as stable as possible and create an optimal environment for recovery while you sleep.

Meal 1	P + V + F
Meal 2	P + V + F
Meal 3	P+ V + C
Meal 4	P+ V + C
Meal 5	P+ V + C
Meal 6	P + V + F

Demographic Profile: Those wishing to gain muscle or 'bulk' in a healthy way

Recommendation: Combine meals into a PVCF combination. Consider packaging a PVCCF meal post-workout. Increase indulgence meals to 2–3 times per week. Be patient as your body adapts to more food, especially those that are nutrient dense.

Warning: The more you stick to your strategy of fueling your body with strategic power foods, the greater ability your body will have to cut body fat while holding onto precious lean muscle tissue. Be careful not to fall into the mentality that you can eat whatever you want since you're "bulking." I will cover bulking/re-framing in a later chapter.

Demographic Profile: Those sensitive to carbohydrates or who experience bloating often.

Recommendation: Stick to PVF meals for the majority of the time, or utilize a PVcf meal (half peak range of carbs and fats, so 10–15 grams of carbs or 4–6 grams of fat) to help your body reduce the amount of carbohydrates you intake at one time, while still benefiting from the lower energy intake.

Warning: By reducing your carbohydrate intake, you may be prone to really bloating and feeling "fluffy" when you do let down your guard and eat carbs, particularly highly-refined carbohydrates. Make this attempt only if you are committed to 1-2 indulgence meals per week (sometimes you need to cut the indulgence meal for the first few weeks to get your body rolling).

Demographic Profile: Those wishing to cut body fat quickly and be in utter control (Note: this is a DIET mentality—not a lifestyle. You should default to lifestyle structure with more planned carbs at the conclusion of this phase).

Recommendation: This is what I personally use often, which is called the "Intuition Shred." This is where you have your P and V at every meal, but you ask yourself whether you need a C or an F when it's time to eat. If you feel weak and lacking energy, have a C. If you feel hungry and need satiety, have an F. It's that simple. If you are feeling just fine, you may "strip" the C or the F from the meal and only enjoy a PV meal. It is best to consider stripping a *maximum* of two meals in a day, with your main meals (Meals 1, 3, and 5) keeping the integrity of a PVC or PVF meal, making Meals 2, 4, or 6 the meals you may consider stripping if you feel well enough (you don't have to.)

Warning: The "Intuition Shred" as I call this approach takes an extreme amount of discipline and honesty with yourself. Seek to comply, not justify. Your body can take more than you think. Most people can't last over 2-3 weeks of this as it takes much mental exertion. When you burn out, please default to a structured plan instead of going ballistic. This takes great control and mental focus and you will do best if you are coached through it for accountability.

There are many additional strategies and methods to structure your own PFL:

Carb Cycling: Consult with Body Buddies Coaches

Ketogenic Plan: Consult with Body Buddies Coaches

Endurance Sports/Athletic Plan: Consult with Body Buddies Coaches

Pregnancy/Lactation: Consult with Body Buddies Coaches, or purchase Power Foods for Two: A Lifestyle for the Pregnant Woman on www.body-buddies.com.

Conclusion

The PFL principles give you a lingo and basic methodology for meal combinations that can be adapted to any particular nutritional need. Experiment with your body and you can eventually identify food allergies you may never have known you have, and find the optimal way to fuel yourself and maximize the look and functioning of your body. It's an amazing thing to experience the many *"a-ha! moments"* the PFL will give you.

11

Meal Timing

When did we go from babies who were fed at regular intervals to growing up and neglecting to be regimented about the nutrition that goes into our adult bodies? Though it makes sense to say *"life gets in the way," "we're too busy,"* and *"we just have other priorities,"* let's stop using those justification statements.

Are we living just to die? As soon as we cross a threshold of age, are we no longer important? Should our health be placed on the back burner? I hardly think so, and though on a cognitive level you probably agree with me, putting good habits in place is tough, isn't it?! That's okay. That's why we focus primarily on *implementing the principles* of the PFL into your life, and less on rigid perfection.

Your body is a miraculous machine that needs to be fed consistently throughout the day. Although you may initially feel the PFL recommendations are too often and for too much food (most people feel this way when they start), your body will quickly adapt to the frequent schedule of eating—it takes about a week or two.

You will soon begin to realize that a satisfied feeling is far better than a full feeling. You should only be eating to this level of satisfied. After some time, your body will begin to tell you when it's time to eat and you won't need to pay such rigid attention to the clock anymore. You may experience new propensities to fuel yourself, which can be odd if you formerly followed the typical American diet—skip breakfast, eat a big lunch, drink soda all afternoon, then gorge on dinner and snacks all evening.

When you follow this new strategy of eating, your body will begin to function, feel, and look much healthier.

Breaking any habits and forming new patterns of behavior takes only a few weeks of focused effort before it becomes much easier and requires less focus. No matter your age or background, you have the ability to control your new schedule of eating. However, you must first believe it. Until then, I'll believe it for you and you can rely on me.

When to Eat

The timing of your meals depends entirely on your personal schedule. As everyone has a body clock dictated by their schedule, it's important not to use the legendary "rules" to which many cling (like the saying "don't eat after 7 p.m." This is bogus to me. There is no definition for whom that rule could be beneficial. If my client was working a graveyard shift, or staying up late for circumstances outside their control, that statement seems extremely unrealistic). Instead, try using the guidelines below to adapt as life happens and your schedule fluctuates from day to day and week to week.

Guideline #1: Eat Meal 1 within 1 hour of waking.
Get that metabolism going first thing! If you're always in a hurry, you will do well to bulk prep a breakfast from the *Power Foods Lifestyle Recipe Books* to quickly grab and run out the door.

Guideline #2: Eat every 2.5–3 hours following Meal 1.
Above all else, listen to your body. You should not have a growling stomach for long as that's a message from your body that it's in danger of slowing its metabolism to preserve energy. Give it food before this happens! I'd like you to always stay ahead of hunger. Depending on your schedule, you might need more or less frequent meals. The key is to do your best with what you have, not to follow a rigid set of principles that cannot be met every single day. Adapt, adapt, adapt.

Guideline #3: Eat a meal one hour before your workout.
If you're planning to workout upon waking, it may be beneficial for you to have 1/3 the size of a meal, or experiment with a little bit of protein, carbs, and/or fats. You might also feel better working out on an empty stomach. I usually have my clients try just one macronutrient category before their workout for a few days, then change it up. We know after 1-2 weeks what they feel best on, and can quickly help them feel their best while losing fat, and help them avoid nausea that can often occur if an individual works out on an empty stomach. If your workout falls after

any number of meals, you will learn to set your pre-workout meal time, then plan backwards until you know your meal intervals for the day. If you have a fluctuating workout schedule like me, this takes just a few moments of thought each night to plan for the next day.

Guideline #4: Eat your final meal 1.5–2 hours before bed.
Notice how I didn't say "Meal 6?" I said "final meal." Let's say you go to bed a bit early one night. Does that mean you need to force-feed yourself and get that sixth meal in? Not at all. Remember, you are trying to preserve the environment of your body, not treat it like a bank account that needs a particular number of calories and macronutrients daily.* This means that depending on the window of time you are awake, you may eat a different number of meals each day.

What if you need to pull a late night? Then you will most likely eat more than six meals. Continue to eat a balanced meal at regular feeding intervals of 2.5-3 hours. Unless you need the energy or you're in a mental fog, PVF meals will be best for helping optimize your blood sugar when in a fat loss phase.

When working with a coach to repair your metabolism or preparing for bodybuilding competitions, this principle may shift. Talk to your coach if you have a question about this.

Benefits of Eating Smaller, Frequent Meals
It can feel odd to think of eating so often when you're used to eating larger meals only one to three times per day. I am often told by new clients that it "seems like so much food!" That is, until the 1-2 week adjustment period is over, then they begin to experience what I've been telling them about. Many people have never listened to their bodies to know when it is signaling hunger. Achieving this is a great triumph as the typical American's metabolism is so sluggish and behavior so unregulated that true hunger is a feeling very foreign.

The statement that smaller, more frequent meals "work" or" don't work" for fat loss has been a controversy in the nutrition world for years. As I research and observe trends of the many people who pass through the Body Buddies coaching program, I ascertain that the benefit of smaller, more frequent meals for sedentary populations is mostly psychological, while for more active and athletic populations, mostly physiological. With that said, eating at the PFL recommended frequency has multiple benefits that can enhance your body's health and amplify the fat loss process, no matter which level of fitness you currently enjoy. Let's go through them one by one:

1. Many studies show that people who eat smaller, more frequent meals tend to eat fewer calories in a day than people who eat three larger meals.

- Eating frequently helps prevent you from overconsuming at your next meal, which typically happens when you are ravenous from going too long without eating and your blood sugar has dropped (we'll cover that in point 3). If you're not overconsuming and you do well at sticking to the PFL portion size for your body, your caloric deficit may increase consistently over time as your metabolism builds and functions more optimally. When coupled with exercise, appropriate caloric deficits lead to a need for your body to rid itself of stored energy, or body fat.

- If you eat at 7 a.m. and then wait until 12 or 1 p.m. to eat again, you're probably very hungry by the time the next meal time arrives. Your blood sugar has dropped, your head begins to pound, and you find yourself more irritable than usual. This is a typical physiological response to low blood sugar. In addition to these pre-eating consequences are the post-eating consequences: you most likely over-fill your plate and eat more than you should because you are so hungry. You allow yourself this overconsumption because of the amount of time that has passed between meals.

This causes your blood sugar to rise, and insulin rushes to capture and transport glucose for active use, preventing you from going into a potentially deadly hyperglycemic coma. While insulin secretion saves us all from this fate, there is a problem that prevents fat loss: when the storage hormone, insulin, is secreted from your pancreas, any glucose that is not actively needed or can be stored for later use as glycogen triggers your fat cells to convert the molecules into fatty acids and store them. When insulin levels are elevated, fatty acids aren't allowed to be mobilized and burned off for energy. This is counterproductive when you're trying to decrease body fat.

It's very important not to skip any meals so you can keep your blood sugar level fluctuations as minimal as possible. Make every effort to fuel your body regularly, and try not to allow your stomach to growl in hunger. Those hunger pains and noises are warnings that your body has run out of fuel and is transitioning into a state of stress. When your body is stressed, it shifts the focus from that of nutrient-absorbing, energy-producing, and fat-blasting to metabolism-slowing, nutrient-preserving, and fat-blast-halting.

- I don't know too many people—sedentary or athletic in fitness level—who have absolutely unbreakable willpower to turn down yummy doughnuts or cookies that are sitting in the break room at work when they're hungry. Fueling your body with nutrient-rich foods helps balance your blood sugar. This gives you extra willpower to say 'no' by promoting biochemical balance in your body. Perhaps you will also achieve greater mental balance by being able to remind yourself, it's okay—I get to eat my meal in another 45 minutes. If I'm still hungry after my next meal, I can go ahead and have the cookie.

• Most people who are serious about making a change in their body find they have the motivation and desire to turn down non-strategic temptations after getting a balanced PFL meal in their body. They focus on what they *can* have, rather than what they *can't* have. This helps prevent overconsumption and binges that prevent your body from changing and getting healthier.

• Eating frequently brings psychological and emotional satisfaction. Wouldn't you much rather eat five or six times per day rather than three? Putting food in your mouth is fun, so if you have the time, having a meal every 2.5–3 hours can be the very thing that helps you compartmentalize your day and be more productive.

2. "Increased meal frequency appears to have a positive effect on various blood markers of health, particularly LDL cholesterol, total cholesterol, and insulin."[9] I have observed this change in many of my clients' results from health checks, and always look forward to texts and emails from former clients who continue with the lifestyle. They describe the look on their doctors' faces when seeing the changes in cholesterol, blood pressure, triglycerides, and body fat. Those messages make me throw my fist in the air in triumph. People every day are changing their lives! It's your turn!

• Smaller, more frequent meals help you better manage Type 1 and Type 2 Diabetes. With more structure and systematic eating times, you can quickly adapt to the amount of insulin you will need as you learn your body's response to particular PVC and PVF meals that are in the peak range best for your body and your fitness level. Learn more about Diabetes management with the PFL in the chapter on Miscellaneous Goals.

• High Cholesterol impacts many. The result of many people's continuation of

---

[9] http://www.fda.gov/Food/GuidanceRegulation/GuidanceDocumentsRegulatoryInformation/LabelingNutrition/ucm064872.htm

the principles of the PFL include lowered cholesterol numbers. Since this book was first published in 2013, I've received numerous emails from individuals who have never been a one-on-one client, but who have seen dramatic changes in their bodies through the PFL methodology. Medication is not always the answer. I believe strongly in the power of strategic nutrition, and hope you will soon join me in watching your body change for the better.

Cholesterol has two forms: dietary cholesterol, which comes from animal sources like meat, poultry, and full-fat dairy, and cholesterol that is produced by your liver. This happens when you put Trans fats and high sugar intakes in your body. You may be hesitant to eat animal protein, egg yolks, or full-fat dairy because of what you have believed about cholesterol. However, the majority of people don't need to eliminate these food products from their lives as dietary cholesterol is not the villain here. Your goal should be to keep oils with Trans fats out of your body in addition to high sugar foods. These are the primary culprits for producing the wax-like substance that builds up and clogs your arteries.

• Increased meal frequency can help with insulin resistance, which is when cells in your body lose their reactive ability to insulin. This results in increased blood sugar levels. Many people experience insulin resistance without being aware of it, and the exact cause is not completely understood in current academia. However, the greatest school of thought to which I add my observations are the following:

• Excess body weight
• Physical inactivity
• Long periods of yo-yo dieting
• Frequent consumption of refined carbohydrates in excess

Which came first, the chicken or the egg? It's a rhetorical question without a real answer as you can argue either way. I feel the same way about insulin resistance and belly fat (visceral fat—the most dangerous type of fat as it surrounds organs such as the liver, pancreas, and intestines.) Does a person gain excess weight which results in insulin resistance? Or does a person develop insulin resistance which results in increased belly fat? I don't know if the answer really matters. What matters is that you immediately begin putting in place the changes in food choices, food combinations, meal timing, and portions that will help your body begin evolving to a state of efficient function.

- Increasing your meal frequency can help eliminate any nutrient deficiencies you might have. Fueling your body at a consistent and steady rate, especially with a variety of vegetables at every meal, gives your body the time and energy for carriers to absorb important nutrients (power fats are essential for absorbing vitamins A, D, E, and K). Consistency in fueling yourself is what helps your body get the vitamins and minerals it needs to correct the outward manifestation of nutritional deficiencies (loss of hair, bruising, dark circles under the eyes, etc.).

3. Eating small, frequent meals leads to increased fat loss as your blood sugar levels are more stable than when going long periods of time without food.

- When you go too long between meals, your blood sugar levels begin to drop. When your blood sugar is in this lowered state, your metabolism (think of it as the total speed of all bodily chemical processes, which include digestion and energy production) slows to preserve the limited amounts of glucose, and will even call upon your liver to break down glycogen (previously stored energy from carbohydrates) to get more glucose in your blood. Eating a large meal after going without food will take your blood sugar from this lower state and cause it to suddenly jump to an elevated state due to the influx of glucose. This is known as an insulin "spike."

Your metabolism, which can slow when in a state of preservation, is now caught off guard and takes time to adjust to the influx. Depending on the amount and composition of the foods in your meal, your body could go into "storage mode." This is due to insulin being secreted by your pancreas to help with the absorption of so much energy in your blood stream—insulin will signal your body to pull it all in for use or storage!

Sudden fluctuations in blood sugar can make you very irritable as well and cause you to "crash" later if your meal consisted of lots of sugar and highly-refined carbohydrates. Nobody likes to be around a "grumpy gills," as Dora in *Finding Nemo* would say. Simply for the sake of the happiness of people around you, choose to eat small, frequent meals to keep your blood sugar levels more stable.

Skipping Breakfast

You might find yourself skipping breakfast for several reasons:

- You feel it makes you hungrier sooner. When you have a busy life and much to do, taking time to eat seems more an interruption than a necessity.
- You forget. When eating in the beginning of the day isn't a programmed habit and you're in a rush, it simply doesn't happen.
- You feel guilty about overeating the night before. You may have had too much to eat, or a snack you didn't plan on, so feel you should skip a meal in order to "make up" the extra calories.

When you wait to have your first meal, you might reduce the number of hours that your metabolism could be running optimally. If you have a fairly average daily waking time of 6 a.m. to 11 p.m. and are waiting until noon to eat, you may be narrowing yourself to a window of as little as ten to eleven hours during which your body is actually working to break down, absorb, transport, and digest the nutrients you're putting into your body.

You might eat a larger meal within that eleven-hour window under the impression that it's fine, since you're still under your daily caloric goal. Unfortunately, your body doesn't function optimally under this method of being fueled. You're expecting it to do too much in too little time. Your body simply doesn't have the time to go through all of the processes it needs in order to utilize the food as fuel, so it ends up keeping some around for storage. The key to getting your body functioning normally—metabolizing all of the fuel you put in your body and utilizing it for energy and nutrients—is to eat smaller, more frequent meals.

Changing this habit in your life can have long-lasting effects on your composition and the way you function each day. Breakfast is about getting necessary glucose and vitamins in your body to aid brain function and energy production. When you change your mindset to think of food as fuel, you'll stop neglecting the critical starting point each day by eating your first meal.

Eating with your Workout in Mind

In order to create the best environment for a body composition-shifting workout (less body fat, more muscle), be sure to have a meal approximately one hour before you plan to start your exercise. This gives your body the fuel it needs, but allows a good amount of digestion to occur in order to avoid getting an upset stomach during your workout.

Here is a method you can try to make sure your pre-workout meal is spot on: plan your workout time each night before going to bed, then plan your meal times backward from one hour prior to the workout start time.

Meal 1. Doing so will fuel your workout with the nutrients and energy you need to be effective.

Example: Bob—wakes at 6 a.m., works out at 5 p.m., and goes to sleep at 11 p.m.

Waking: 6 a.m.
Meal 1: 7 a.m.
Meal 2: 10 a.m.
Meal 3: 1:00 p.m.
Meal 4: 4:00 p.m. (one hour prior to workout)
Workout: 5:00 pm-6:00 pm
Meal 5: 6:30 p.m. (within one hour of finishing his workout)
Meal 6: 9:00 p.m.
Bedtime: 11:00 p.m.

What if you are an early morning exerciser? This is tough as there are so many factors that make a difference. If you want assurance that you are employing the best option for you, please be sure to schedule a consultation (conducted via Skype or FaceTime) with one of the Body Buddies coaches. Additionally, please remember the PFL is a system of principles for any number of goals, whether it's cutting (reducing) body fat or gaining muscle (please refer to the chapter for Miscellaneous Goals).

All bodies are not created the same, so use the following guidelines as a starting point, then use your intuition and observations to listen to what your body tells you to tweak.

Cardio Only Workout: I recommend doing this only 3-4 times max per week, and on a fasted stomach first thing after waking up and drinking 2 cups of ice cold water. No need to chase the cardio with a protein shake, just eat within 30 minutes following the session to keep your metabolism going at an increased rate.

There are conflicting academic studies on whether performing cardio on an empty stomach is more beneficial to body fat loss than afterwards—I think it's important to take into account the nature of the cardio. For steady-state cardio in an aerobic threshold (60-70% of your maximum heart rate)[10], an empty stomach should be fine. For a more energy-requiring cardio workout with intervals or even High-Intensity Interval Training (HIIT), which should be performed at 75-85% of your maximum heart rate, you may amplify your fat loss by eating a small amount of food prior to the workout. I have had clients try any one of the macronutrient categories prior to their HIIT workouts and feel good and lose body fat over the course of our training. Again, it's about finding what feels good for your body. Try something like the following:

- Protein: 2 oz. turkey breast, or ½ protein shake
- Carbs: 1 serving of any one of my Power Foods snack bars/cookies or 1/3 c. oats with honey
- Fats: 1–2 Tbsp. raw nuts or 1 Tbsp. 100% natural peanut butter

Resistance Training + Cardio Workout: Eat 1/3–1/2 of Meal 1 immediately upon waking, or drink ½ a protein shake with ¼-½ c carbs with it (try Grapenuts®, rolled oats, unsweetened Bran flakes, or Wheat Chex®). If you eat 1/3–1/2 of Meal 1 prior to exercise, eat the other ½ –2/3 within 30 minutes of finishing your post-workout shake (if you're training hard enough for muscle toning/growth). If you only drank ½ a protein shake prior to the workout, drink the other ½ upon completion of the resistance training. Meal 1 should follow 15-30 minutes later.

A post-workout shake can be important to drink (15–30 grams of protein) within 30-60 minutes of finishing your workout. This time period right after exercise is known as the "Anabolic Window." This is when you can best replenish and refuel the muscles and depleted glycogen in your body. This helps you to recover more quickly, and gives your body the fuel it needs as you are working to change your shape. Though the Anabolic Window is a term used heavily in bodybuilding and athletic performance circles, this is a principle of nutrition that I believe all who exercise rigorously should adopt. I have worked with many clients who don't wish to use, or have an allergy to, protein powder. Is this a make-or-break principle? Not at all. If you are one of these people, simply be sure to eat your next PVC meal soon after the workout.

Endurance Activity: If you'll be spending more than 60 minutes in continuous aerobic activity, it's best to focus on carbohydrate-based foods with a little protein. Try ½ a banana with ½ Tbsp. peanut butter, then re-fuel with something similar in portion every 45-60 minutes for the duration of the activity, with a PVC (protein-veggie-carb) meal as soon as you can eat after the activity.

---

[10] To find max heart rate, simply subtract your age from 220 as the easiest method. For example, if you are 40 years old, take 220 and subtract 40. Your max heart rate is 180 bpm.

Don't Fear Food Post-Workout

During many years of my teenage and early-twenties life, I had a skewed mindset about eating post-workout. I had just done all of that work to burn so many calories—why on earth would I put more food and calories in my body? It didn't make sense to me when people said I needed to refuel my body. I find that most people looking to lose body fat fall into this mindset as well. It's the "bank account" mentality rather than the "environment" mentality I'm trying to help you learn.

I'd like you to look at it this way: let's think of how much work you just did in breaking your muscles down and expending energy (calories is simply a form of measuring energy.) When you fail to replenish your body with nutrients, it senses that it needs to draw on its own stores to provide that energy. Unfortunately, your body will not just magically turn to your fat storage for this (although that would be nice!).

Only when your body is in a very consistent, predictable state can it stay in fat-burn zone. Additionally, depending on the intensity and duration of exercise you performed, your body may be at a heightened metabolic state for 12-24 hours following your workout. Without fuel, your body won't be able to maximize the increased workload you've given it to make more change happen in your body.

Sounds Great, But I'm Busy

I understand you're a busy person. Eating as frequently as I suggest may not seem overly-appealing to you as it requires some time you'll need to carve out of your schedule. If you aren't used to this kind of an eating routine, it may seem a bit intimidating, or even impossible. You have a job, meetings, kids, errands, hobbies, and other never-ending obligations.

Take it with a grain of salt—these are just excuses. You have 24 hours in a day just like everyone else. You have to eat just like everyone else. It's time to examine what's holding you back and seek to eliminate negativity and rationalization from your mind. Surely you can take a few extra minutes to take some food from a plastic bag and put it into your mouth, chew, and swallow. If you knew that eating according to these recommendations would help you lose weight and keep it off as you keep the habit, wouldn't you be willing to juggle things in your life slightly? One of my favorite saying is, "If nothing changes, nothing changes." Until you change your habits and behaviors from their current state, your body and health will not change from their current state.

Adapting to the PFL principles takes planning. It's very possible for you to make this lifestyle work, though you may need to be a bit more creative and thorough in your food prep (see Chapter 17 on Helpful Tidbits) or get custom coaching to aid you in the process. Remember that you are worth the extra effort! Unless you take care of yourself, how can you be effective in your job or hobbies and deliver quality performance? Think about your life and how much better you'll be able to perform your daily tasks if you're feeling energized and healthy. You'll be a better husband, wife, father, mother, boss, employee, friend, co-worker, and neighbor. Positive results work like a magnet to attract other positive results. Forget the fear and discomfort of trying this new lifestyle, and just go for it!

Keep in mind that your PFL meals don't have to be elaborate, hot meals that are eaten at your table with silverware and a napkin on your lap. If I had a dollar for every time I've grabbed a container of previously-prepared meals out of the fridge, thrown it in my purse, and run out the door to get on my way, I'd probably have a few thousand bucks. Success in this lifestyle requires you to plan ahead so that your chaotic life doesn't get in the way of you achieving your goals and fueling your body for prime energy.

Conclusion

This lifestyle comes down to planning and preparation. As you train your body to expect nourishing food at frequent intervals, you may see many aspects of your health improve, including your psychological relationship with food. Seek to gain consistency in all you do, as therein lies the secret to mastery and achievement. Don't expect perfection of yourself, but strive to make progress, plan ahead, and overcome obstacles that arise through strategy. You can improve on small elements daily. You can begin putting your health at the priority number it should be—after all, you can only be your best and help others when you're feeling good about yourself both inside and out.

12
Portion Sizes

I absolutely hate being hungry, don't you? In fact, fear of being hungry is one of the greatest mental obstacles I've had to work through in order to better discipline how my body looks and functions. For many years, fear caused me to drown in this cycle:

deprivation > binge > purge/over-exercise > repeat

When I learned to fuel my body regularly instead of deprive myself as I tried to lose body fat, I found that I was able to start controlling my binging behavior. Can you relate to those times that you feel out of control, yet you can't stop eating? It feels awful, doesn't it? You know that you should stop, but it's just too hard to say "no." The motion of hand-to-mouth feels so good and your taste buds beckon for more, and more, and more.

One of the negative results of these actions is that you might awful about yourself after the overconsumption. You feel the lack of self-control. You feel the frustration when you try on your clothes or look in the mirror. Any form of overeating on a consistent basis will prevent you from achieving the body shape you want and promote negative feelings about yourself. These are all no good—life is too short to be experiencing this negativity! I want to help you change this about yourself, so we're going to learn the strategies and tricks to preventing the behavior from ever occurring.

Do Not Starve Yourself

Most people's natural impulse when trying to lose weight is to skimp on food, or withhold it altogether. I've worked with people who suffer from anorexia, where withholding food has little to no connection to their body, but is a form of control and superiority over their actions. While anorexia is more of a psychological challenge, I have found that nutritional education can aid the process of healing as the individual uses logic and education to empower their daily decisions, rather than willpower and psychological control alone.

For those who aren't dealing with Anorexia, but are simply trying to lose weight (body fat), skimping too much on food is actually a very counterproductive way to lose weight. Most people I work with are in disbelief when they see their first week of food and how much I expect them to eat. Oftentimes it is more than they have been eating for years. In their minds, they feel that if I'm going to help them reach their goals, they should be eating fewer calories, and even smaller portion sizes than I am assigning them. I smile with each new client who voices these concerns because I understand where they're coming from, and the myth about weight loss they have come to believe: the myth that deprivation is the key to weight loss. This is not true, Body Buds. It's simply not true.

In order for your metabolism to begin running more efficiently, you must put 'fuel' in there to begin with. As you do so, your body can begin to work like a machine. It will absorb nutrients and burn through the energy from the food you put in your body. Just as a car cannot run without gasoline in its tank, your body will not get you very far nor feel powerful without adequate fuel.

I ask for your trust and willingness to open your mind as you begin following the PFL. Yes, it's going to feel like you're eating a lot, and often, perhaps going against our natural impulses of withholding food as you may have done in the past. But fueling your body is good. The structure of the food combinations is strategic. When you are eating the right kinds of foods—power foods—you have the luxury of eating a much greater volume of food than you ever could on processed and refined garbage. I know it's new to you and even scary to try this. I know it's a bizarre thought to consider feeling better, and embracing a body with less body fat for life. But I also want you to realize this act of building habits will extend beyond food and impact other parts of your life—this discipline will help you evolve as a person for the rest of your life. It is far better to do this the scientific and healthful way, instead of doing some crash-and-burn escapade that will land you physically and emotionally exhausted, with a damaged metabolism that can take years to repair.

Benefits of Portion Size Awareness

Eating proper portion sizes in strategic food combinations provides your body with nutrients and energy it needs for day-to-day function. The PFL principles will help prevent you from giving your body too much fuel—particularly carbohydrates—which can disturb the fat-burning environment.

Eating according to your portion sizes will also benefit you psychologically—one of my favorite parts of the PFL. Regularly fueling yourself gives you the logic to deflect any feelings of *I'm hungry, I need to eat.* You can be confident that your body is fueled, and you don't need more food. It's at that point you can identify what has triggered your appetite (or 'fixations,' as I would rather call what most people call 'cravings') by using principles you learned in Chapter 2 on Mental Discipline. After identifying what has triggered your urge to eat, you can logically process yourself through your fixation and address the real issue.

Were you feeling extremely stressed, sad, disappointed, hurt, or lonely? Often your "eat now" urges are associated with an emotion that stands completely independent from true physical hunger.

After each meal, you should feel nourished and satisfied, which is a different feeling than what you might feel following Thanksgiving dinner. Your meal should never cause your stomach to bloat terribly or even 'pooch out.' You may or may not feel slightly hungry by the time your next meal rolls around, but it's important you eat—especially in the initial weeks of training your body and teaching it this new way of functioning. By doing this, you completely avoid true hunger and the feeding frenzies that can result from it. As a result, your hormones stay in balance and you prevent any sudden surges of insulin.

You might wonder if I'm talking about force feeding yourself—definitely not. The PFL is about learning to pay attention to your body and listening to its cues. However, that experience and knowledge won't come until you've trained your body to know what it needs. In my custom coaching programs one-on-one and group 8-week Challenges, I encourage people to eat according to their pre-planned meal times for the initial 8 weeks. After that time period, your body will be ready to tell you when it needs food and when it doesn't. You can then begin running off hunger cues to pace your eating.

Your Eyes Are Often Bigger Than Your Stomach

When you see a food that visually stimulates your sensory neurons, a pleasure point suddenly goes off in your brain. You subconsciously begin tasting the food and preparing for the bliss that will occur as your taste buds relish in the flavor and textures—all before you ever take a bite.

Because of these triggers, most people tend to serve themselves a bit too much and wind up eating more energy calories than their body needs. This triggers the release of our good friend insulin, which helps signal the transportion of nutrients to your body's active needs. Well, when there are enough nutrients to fuel your body, what happens to the excess? Insulin is what triggers the storage of fatty acids broken down in your blood stream to be stored as fat when there is no need for active use or storage. That extra serving of food can quickly be stored as 'fluffy little pillows' along your waistline, hips, and thighs.

It will take time to get used to how a "normal" PFL meal looks. After you have trained yourself on PFL portions, you might be baffled by restaurants as you notice just how big those portion sizes are. You might see how quickly the dining and fast food industries have changed the size of America's waistlines.

Beginning to Measure

Mastering the ability to control your portions is critical to your success in beginning a new and healthy lifestyle. For the first few weeks following the PFL, I suggest you use a food scale[11] and measuring cups to weigh or measure the majority of your foods. Weighing and measuring your food should not become an obsessive behavior that you continue; instead, measuring your food is a key step in training your eyes to recognize proper portion sizes for your body type and goal.

A frequent obstacle in controlling your portions can be the crockery companies. They stock store shelves with beautifully designed—but large— dishes. As a result, you eat more than you need, often without even realizing it. This is simply due to the principle of perspective. I remember getting bothered with my mom when I was younger as she served the boys in the family on larger dishes than the girls. I wanted as much food as them! Hindsight says she understood much better than I the principle of the dishes we eat in relationship to how much we eat, and was looking out for me—teaching me proper portion sizes. I now happily enjoy eating off the smaller plates when I visit my parents in my hometown.

Try this exercise to better understand what I mean. Scoop out ½ cup of cottage cheese and put it in the middle of a large plate. Doesn't the serving of cottage cheese look tiny compared to the large circular plate around it? Like hardly anything is there? Refer to the figure below.

Now scoop out the same serving of cottage cheese (½ cup) and place

---

[11] Food scales can be purchased at fairly inexpensive prices of $20-$50 at your local Walmart or Target. While I recommend that you eventually leave the scales and use approximate sizes instead, initially measuring is very good training for those who have never learned about proper portions.

it on a small plate. Does this
serving of cottage cheese still
look tiny compared to the larger
plate? No. It fills the whole
plate, giving it the appearance
of being much more than the
cottage cheese in the center of
the large plate.

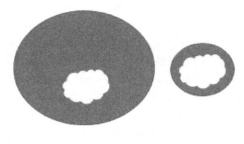

Visual cues are important in triggering your mind to feel satisfied with the amount of food you're giving it. Make a goal to downsize your dishes, or be aware of the psychological result of the dish sizes you use.

A Few Techniques

Portion sizes can be even more difficult to control when dining out. One strategy you can employ to keep your portions under control is to order a smaller-sized option if it's available—like a half salad instead of full, or 6-oz. sirloin instead of 12. If only large portions are available, be proactive. It can be unwise to trust yourself to stop eating when you've reached a feeling of having enough. That feeling usually comes 3-5 minutes after you *should* have stopped eating. In addition to this, the social atmosphere and succulent tastes can entice you to eat more than you know you should.

When you order, ask your server to bring a to-go box to the table when he or she brings your meal. Before you ever begin eating, divide your meal into more PFL appropriate portions. Place the remainder of your meal in the box, and set it under the table where it's out of sight. This is a simple strategy that makes a difference in the long run as it becomes a habit.

Another trick I learned is from the incredible book *Mindless Eating* by Brian Wansink, Ph.D., is to never eat out of an open bag. It's so easy to go in for handful after handful without realizing how much you are eating. This can also easily occur as you are often busy multi-tasking—watching TV, checking social media, reading the newspaper, or texting on your cell phone. Instead of this disastrous eating habit, serve one portion into a small dish or plastic bag. Utilizing this strategy will ensure you practice self-control and eat the correct portion for the optimum fat burning environment in your body—no more, no less.

What is Your Portion Size?

As this is a lifestyle, not a diet program, it is very important that you learn what works best with your body. Try these suggestions initially and monitor your body on a weekly basis. Always eat a balanced meal of each of the suggested power foods—simply increase or decrease the portion size of those foods with each meal depending on how full or hungry you feel. This is called keeping "meal integrity." If you have any question at all about the application of these principles and initial guidelines for your body, please schedule a consultation with one of the Body Buddies coaching team—we are here to help and take the guesswork out of your lifestyle change.

Step One: Estimate your total daily calorie consumption

Body Buds, it is nearly impossible for anyone, myself included, to give a perfectly sound definition of how many calories you should or shouldn't eat for weight loss. Gender and age make a difference, as well as current activity level. With that said, use the list below to get a ballpark range of numbers of calories to eat. Please do not think these are "golden" numbers as all bodies are different and exceptions always apply.

Sedentary Definition: You rarely exercise. You sit all day long. Walking up the stairs winds you. This may be due to habit or disability. You don't particularly like the thought of exercise.

Sedentary Man: 1,700 calories daily
Sedentary Woman: 1,200 calories daily

Semi-Active Definition: You exercise 2-3 times per week with a moderate intensity. You work out because you know you should, and you occasionally enjoy it.

Semi-Active Man: 2,000 calories daily
Semi-Active Woman: 1,400 calories daily

Active Definition: You exercise 5-7 times per week and focus on pushing yourself harder every time. You love the feel of being active and being sore from your workouts.

Active Man: 2,400 calories daily
Active Woman: 1,600 calories daily

Step Two: Find out the peak range per meal for each macronutrient

The next step is to take your total number of calories for the day and apply it to the percentage of calories coming from these macronutrients. If you follow the basic PFL to its specific recommendations, 30-40% of your daily calories will be contributed by protein, 30-40% by carbohydrates, and 20-40% by fats. These ballparks are for slow and steady weight loss, correcting nutrient deficiencies, and combatting insulin resistance. Different ranges may be used for various populations as additional PVC/PVF combinations are used later on.

If you feel you will become flustered by the math, simply skip over the equations below and head to the next section. However, I would like you to try and read through it at least once, doing your best to understand and think through the process. This is about you learning—the thought processes here should help you begin to understand how over time, this methodology will help free your mind from calorie counting and, instead, help you think in terms of portions and meal types.

Remember how protein and carbohydrates each have 4 calories per gram, whereas fat has 9 calories per gram? Let's use this information to then find the total amount of grams per macronutrient that you should be eating. As this is a tricky area for most people, I'll walk you through it using a semi-active woman as the example:

Protein: 30-40%
4 calories per gram

Total calories = 1,400   1,400 x 0.35 = 490 calories from protein

Next, we take 490 calories and divide it by 4 calories to arrive at the total number of grams.

490 / 4 = 122.5 grams of protein per day

As the Power Foods Lifestyle has approximately six meals in which you need to eat protein, you would then take 122.5 and divide that by 7 to arrive at a good estimation of protein to eat at each of your six meals. Why 7? Aren't you dividing the protein by six meals? Yes, but we need to account for the residual protein grams that will be contributed from Power Carbs and Power Fats.

122.5 / 7 = 17.5 grams of protein per meal

Do you have to hit 17.5 grams on the spot with each meal? No. This number simply gives you an approximate ball park. Try to hit anywhere from 5 fewer to 5 greater. A semi-active woman's protein peak range would then be 12.5-22.5 grams per meal.

Carbohydrates: 30-40%
4 calories per gram
Total calories = 1,400   1,400 x 0.35 = 490 calories from carbs

Next, we take 490 calories and divide it by 4 calories to arrive at the total number of grams.

$$490 / 4 = 122.5 \text{ gram of carbs per day}$$

As the Power Foods Lifestyle starts with approximately four meals in which you need to eat carbs in PVC meals, you would then take 122.5 and divide that by 5 to arrive at a good estimation of carbs to include in each of your four PVC meals. Why 5? Aren't you dividing the carbs by four meals? Yes, but we need to account for the residual carb grams that will be contributed from Power Protein and Power Fats.

$$122.5 / 5 = 24.5 \text{ grams of carbs per meal}$$

Do you have to hit 24.5 grams on the spot with each meal? No. This number simply gives you an approximate ball park. Try to hit anywhere from 5 fewer to 5 greater. A semi-active woman's carbohydrate peak range would then be 19.5-29.5 grams for each of four PVC meals.

Fat: 20-40%

9 calories per gram

$$\text{Total calories} = 1,400 \qquad 1,400 \times 0.30 = 420 \text{ calories from fat}$$

Next, we take 420 calories and divide it by 9 calories to arrive at the total number of grams.

$$490 / 9 = 54 \text{ grams of fat per day}$$

As the Power Foods Lifestyle starts with the recommendation for two meals in which you need to eat essential fats in PVF meals, you would then take 122.5 and divide that by 3 to arrive at a good estimation of fats to eat in each of the two daily PVF meals. Why 3? Aren't you dividing the fats by two meals? Yes, but we need to account for the residual fat grams that will be contributed from Power Protein and Power Carbs.

$$54 / 3 = 18 \text{ grams of fat per meal}$$

Do you have to hit 18 grams on the spot with each meal? No. That simply gives you an approximate ball park. Try to hit anywhere from 5 fewer to 5 greater. A semi-active woman's fat peak range would then be 13-23 grams for each of her two PVF meals.

Having written thousands of PFL meal plans over the past few years for all kinds of people, activity levels, and histories of health, I will mention that the fat range typically falls a bit lower than the math I just used. I hope showing you the process helps you think on a critical level—however, I typically find in an active application approach that 8-12 grams of fat per PVF meal is the most ideal range for losing body fat.

More Practical Measurements

I hope you weren't overwhelmed by the previous section! It's not imperative to your health that you understand all that mumbo jumbo. What's most important is that you look at the table below and start practicing placing food on your plate that is in these measurements. You will soon learn to gauge the portion size of each of your foods without needing to measure.

	Protein Serving	Carb Serving	Fat Serving	Veggie Serving
Sedentary Woman	3 oz.	1/3 c.	1 Tbsp.	1 c.
Semi- Active Woman	4 oz.	1/2 c.	1 Tbsp.	1 c.
Active Woman	5 oz.	2/3 c.	1.5 Tbsp.	1 c.
Sedentary Man	4 oz.	1/2 c.	1 Tbsp.	1 c.
Semi- Active Man	6 oz.	3/4 c.	1.5 Tbsp.	1 c.
Active Man	6-8 oz.	1 c.	2 Tbsp.	1 c.

Adjusting Portion Sizes

If after two weeks of strict compliance you don't feel like anything is changing in your body, you may decrease the size of your portions, but do not eliminate any one of the macronutrient groups. Keep the meal integrity. The structure of your meals and their PVC/PVF combinations should remain the same. You may simply choose to eat 1/3 cup carbs instead of ½ cup, for example. Don't change any of your meal combinations or the timing of those meals until you have completed an 8-week adjustment period and can then begin manipulating the balance of PVC and PVF meals for your day.

Conclusion

If you are consistently eating small, frequent meals each day, you will be eating frequently enough to avoid the pitfalls of hunger that lead to overeating. Still, mentally guard yourself against this temptation to eat more. It's natural and part of being human. We like to feel satisfied through food. If it becomes a problem that you feel you need help controlling, refer back to the chapters on mental discipline and emotional triggers to examine if your "feelings" of hunger are actually being triggered by something else and are fixations, not cravings.

You have the control and willpower within to discipline yourself. Living the Power Foods Lifestyle should not be torturous—it's freeing. It's not expecting too much of, or being too hard on yourself. This lifestyle involves caring for your body, providing for its needs, and improving your sense of self-control. Seek to remind yourself of that over and over and over. I encourage you to utilize the Body Buddies Podcast, blog, and social media presence in order to keep yourself learning and motivated daily. We're all in the trenches together.

Eating smaller meals more frequently throughout the day will enable your body to heighten its responsiveness to fat loss.

13

Indulgence Meal

H ave you ever watched a *NASCAR* race? The supercharged cars, driven by the best in the world, zoom around the track at lightning speeds. Of course, the cars can't go forever—they have to take a break and idle so the pit crew can do their job. Cars can't run on an empty gas tank, nor can they race on tires without any tread. Stopping momentarily to regroup is crucial to their success.

This is the exact same perspective you need to have about your body.

Many people like to call breaks from their typical nutritional intake "cheat meals." I would like to steer you away from calling them by this name, and direct you to call them "indulgence meals." The verb "cheat" means by definition "to act dishonestly or unfairly in order to gain an advantage." Well guess what, Body Buds? I'm going to teach you how indulging is actually beneficial for your body (when you earn it through compliant behavior to the PFL). Indulgences are planned and earned. They are a part of the plan and an important part of the PFL. Indulgence meals are important both physiologically and psychologically. With this in mind, let's dive into talking about indulgence meals and how you are to approach them.

Eliminate the Fear

When you're disciplined in your eating and doing well at maintaining that resolve, you can easily develop a fear of any kind of indulgence meals or eating outside the plan. In fact, a new eating disorder that has rapidly been gaining attention in these "clean eating" trends is called Orthorexia Nervosa (p.s. I am not a fan of you referring to the PFL as clean eating. I don't believe in dirty eating, so let's instead refer to wholesome or strategic eating). The symptoms of this disorder are when a person has an "unhealthy obsession" with wholesome eating and becomes fixated on food quality and purity.

In all honesty, this is understandable when you go to great lengths to understand just how the food supply works from production to processing and delivery. It can be quite frightening to learn these procedures, then expect yourself to be good, eat perfectly, and make no mistakes in your eating through extremely rigid guidelines. Lack of doing so might result in over-exercising, or increased stringency in eating behaviors. This way of life is not my goal in teaching you about the PFL— rather, my goal is to help you find the balance for yourself, keeping in mind the role of foods in your body.

You may have read those first few paragraphs with wide eyes because you are someone who absolutely loves your indulgence meals—eating anything and everything outside of what you know is best for your body can be a real joy! If this is you, great! The PFL shouldn't make you feel deprived unless you choose to feel that way. Attitude is everything in this effort to discipline your mind and body.

As a human being that needs food to survive, please keep in mind some very important principles that have to do with your indulgence meals.

1. Food should never be feared.
2. Food should never become an obsession or something about which you fantasize.

Food is a wonderful part of our lives that can bring us much happiness and satisfaction, on top of fueling our bodies so we can live. Instead of allowing fear to reside in your mind, work to better understand food and its nutritional properties. With new knowledge, you might more easily find your fears dissipating. Knowledge is extremely empowering when it comes to deciding to live your life free from the constant torment of worry and fear over food. It gives yourself the opportunity to choose logic over emotion.

Logic and education are the #1 methods I used to train my brain and re-program my emotions to have a healthy relationship with food after my "self-mastery moment" in 2012. I feel so happy now that I do not face the love/hate relationship I once had with food. I used to wish I wasn't human so I didn't have to eat. I despised food. It was the enemy because it made me hate myself, as I couldn't control myself around it.

But you know what? I now love and respect food. We have a great relationship. I love the strategic foods, and I love the non-strategic foods. I know when and how to use them to help my body be at its best.

I know that you can overcome anything you're working through as well! We never heal from prior behavior or disorders; instead, we learn to manage our inclinations. We gain confidence from day-by-day choices to live a different way. This gives us momentum to continue onward and create a new life for ourselves. This gives you courage to tip-toe around your triggers as you become aware of them. You can do this!

Psychologically Destructive Practices

It's easy to get sucked into the "food porn" industry where you feast their eyes on ultra-tempting and savory dishes. Social media has become the greatest way to distribute this destructive fad. Pinterest, Facebook, and Instagram are rife with pictures of food that trigger your mind to begin a process that leads to cravings and desire for those foods. I also see thousands of Facebook 'shares' on videos and posts that teach the public how to make confectionary desserts and goodies—they are applauded and worshipped. When you find yourself idolizing food in this way (yes, even healthy foods), you are doing something I call "fixating."

I urge you to pull back from the habit of drooling over these types of pictures. Do not create an environment in your mind where you long for what you are "not allowed" to have. There is nothing positive that results from this practice. All it does is drive home the fact that you are being "deprived," although you are not. Is the practice of keeping foods that may lead your body to being overweight or fraught with disease truly depriving yourself? Or is it liberating yourself?

Perspective is the greatest friend you can keep with you on your journey of adapting to the PFL. It's not about deprivation at all, but enjoyment. As you discipline yourself and keep those indulgence meals and treats out of your typical intake, you will more fully enjoy them at an appropriate time. This is truly the meaning of indulgence, it's not all the time.

Remember that you are not kicking any foods out of your life forever! Heavens no—that's just torture. Instead, you're choosing to put premium fuel into your body 95% of the time, and allowing yourself to splurge the other 5%.

Attitude is everything in training yourself to follow the PFL principles. No, it's not easy. If it were easy, all of America would be jumping on board immediately like they do with every quick weight-loss campaign out there. However, the PFL is the real fix, not the quick fix.

You will only damage your willpower and ability to apply what you are learning as you focus on everything you should not have, or on non-strategic foods more than how wonderful strategic foods you should have. I often remind my clients to reflect back on history, and compare themselves to those who are less fortunate due to war, poverty, or famine. Who are we to complain? Are we starving? Are we sick due to too little food? No. Sometimes we need a very real attitude adjustment when we find ourselves feeling sorry for ourselves.

How often should I indulge?

Many people in the nutrition and diet world promote a cheat, or indulgence day, but I would like to encourage you to stick with one to two indulgence meals per week. When allowed an entire day of indulgence, most people's mentalities of freedom overtake them and they end up completely gorging themselves to the point of being sick. Not only that, but their blood sugar is thrown off so much that the biochemical ability to get back to feeling good takes several days!

If your goal is to lose a significant amount of body fat, I recommend you only plan for one indulgence meal per week. Otherwise, go ahead and plan two indulgence meals. Be sure to plan so you can anticipate your meal of fun (not that eating according to the power foods list isn't fun, but we all enjoy our favorites occasionally).

Planning your indulgence meal will help you stay focused as you adapt to your new lifestyle. When you have something to look forward to, you can often use that as a motivating factor to adhere to what you know is best for your body until then. Many people enjoy planning an indulgence meal for the weekend—either on a Friday, Saturday, or Sunday. It helps them focus and be disciplined during the weekdays.

As you are regularly eating approximately six smaller meals per day, an indulgence meal will actually encompass two meals. For example, if you decided to go out for breakfast for your indulgence meal, this will account for Meals 1 and 2. You should begin eating your regular PFL meals by the time Meal 3 rolls around, and finish the day as normal, beginning to eat your PFL meals again when you feel hungry.

Likewise, if you choose to indulge for a dinner meal, eat your first four meals as usual before indulging for meals 5 and 6. Remember that "saving your calories" will only slow your metabolism and cause your body to hold onto more of what you eat. Repairing and building your metabolism means eating, not going as long as you can without food.

Do not skip any of your other PFL meals, though you may choose to eat smaller portions if you are not truly hungry or ready to eat. You will gain experience to interpret your body's needs, and can know when it needs to simply wait to eat (this takes time and requires training and experience first!). However, when you stick to one indulgence meal and don't allow the windows of non-strategic eating to extend to greater than one meal time, you shouldn't have eaten so much food that you become passive to food the remainder of the day.

Some people feel they are doing so well with their new lifestyle and getting in the habit of making wise food choices that they wish to skip their indulgence meal. This can be fine sometimes, though keep in mind we are trying to develop a lifestyle mentality. There can be a psychological backswing if you push yourself too long without indulging; when you finally allow yourself those foods, you might find it nearly impossible to stop eating. Be wise and choose to indulge once weekly so as to temper the overconsumption that can easily occur through granting yourself "freedom."

Tempering Your Indulgences

Treat your indulgence meal with respect, not a time to go nuts. Any sort of indulgence meal may feel like a desperate attempt to cram every ounce of food within reach into your mouth, drive to every restaurant, and gorge yourself to capacity and beyond. Please guard yourself against these behaviors. You are better than that and can control yourself from a black-or-white, eat-right-or-go-crazy binge. You will feel miserable both physically and mentally. You will feel as though all of your hard work has been undone, and ridicule yourself for being so uncontrolled.

I know this because I've been there and dealt with these behaviors for many years of my own life. The best piece of advice I can give you is to plan your indulgence meals. Eat them slowly, and put your foot down when you feel the signals in your body that you're full. The thought will usually cross your mind: *I really should stop eating now.*

It takes great mental strength to stop, but you can do it. The point that made me realize I must change my behavior was when I realized I could keep repeating this cycle forever, and get nowhere. I was tired of getting nowhere. I decided to push through the "pain" of keeping junk and sweets out of my body except for small portions at infrequent times. My body does not need those things, and neither does yours.

You can become the master of yourself as you work to understand the reasons why you feel so desperate for those foods outside of your power foods. You can find the answers and work to form new mental patterns.

Physiological and Psychological Need

As I mentioned previously, there is both a physiological and psychological need for the indulgence meal. Let's discuss some of these reasons a bit further:

1. Replenish glycogen stores for energy.
Your metabolism needs to be built up and glycogen stores replenished in order to be effective in your next wave of fat loss efforts. Due to lower glycogen levels from

consistent controlled carbohydrate intake, especially if you are being very careful with 2-4 PVC meals, your indulgence meal will not cause you to store fat.

The extra nutrients may cause your body to hold excess water for a day or two, resulting in a higher scale weight, but this will dissipate quickly. Due to this temporary increase, please never weigh yourself within 24 hours of your indulgence meal. If you indulge Saturday night, weigh on Monday or Tuesday morning (always in the morning before having food or water; there are too many metabolic variables that can impact your scale weight—don't give yourself false emotional ammo that "it's not working").

2. Prevent body fat loss plateaus through raising leptin levels.
After restricting your caloric intake consistently for some time, leptin levels in your body begin to lower. Leptin is a hormone that works like a gatekeeper of fat metabolism. When levels are low, we tend to eat more ravenously. When leptin levels are high, we eat with normal signals of hunger and satisfaction. We want to keep leptin levels high if we plan on keeping ourselves and our appetites in control.

Several studies find that leptin levels drop by approximately 50% after about 7 days of restrictive eating—restrictive meaning a minimum of a 400-600 caloric deficit. That means that an indulgence meal one to two times per week is perfect timing to reset your leptin levels. One meal if you're taking more of a moderate approach, and two if you're taking more of a rigid and disciplined approach. Resetting your leptin levels is done with excess calories, most particularly carbohydrates.

Please keep in mind that everyone's leptin levels don't work the same way. The higher the body fat you have, the less quickly your leptin levels drop, making the indulgence meal less of a physiological need, but more of a psychological need and motivating factor to keep you going. The physiological need comes in high demand when you have achieved a lean or less than average body weight; you will need the reset to continue pushing your leanness to new levels as your body naturally fights the lower body fat state.

3. Provide a little bit of "I'm a normal human being" sanity relief.
If you have worked for it the remainder of the week and put aside the temptation for your favorite, but non-strategic foods for that time period, you have earned it! It's quite important for your sanity and making this way of eating a true lifestyle to remove the disciplined mindset for a short time. After all, it is a rare person who is over-consumed enough to put their nose to the grindstone for their whole

life! Food can be a very fun and rewarding part of life, the key is that we temper ourselves and respect the body we have.

Many people find it difficult to indulge as they torture themselves afterward. They think, *"Now I've done it—I've gone and ruined all of my good progress."* They consider themselves weak and feel horrible. They may then take their next dieting to the extreme by either skipping meals, cutting portions, or engaging in excess cardio exercise. These are all the wrong approaches and I caution you to fortify yourself against these thoughts and feelings. You can only do this by further educating yourself on the body mechanisms of glycogen replenishment and hormone resetting. You might also look at several other items:

• Did you earn the meal by adhering to your disciplined approach during the week? If you found yourself cutting corners, taking snitches of non-strategic foods, or not sticking perfectly to your own standard of PFL principles, then you might do better not to take the indulgence meal as you didn't truly earn it.

• Did you stop eating when your body signaled that you were full? If you continued eating past those satisfaction cues, you might examine whether or not you put strategies in place to help you stop. Things like placing a serving in a dish instead of eating from an open bag or asking the waiter or waitress for a to-go box before the meal started. help you better put on the eating brakes. You know yourself better than anyone else, so work to put in place the strategies that will help you not fall victim to yourself. We are each fallible, so do your best to learn from your errors, getting right back in the ball game. Refuse to let any less-than-stellar performance hold you back from making noble efforts in the future!

• Did you plan your indulgence meal? I have had former clients who became very upset when they had to "use" their indulgence meal for an outing or food that wasn't in their forecast. This can happen when you attend banquets, conferences, or attend outings with family or friends. Be very decisive about what classifies as an indulgence meal, versus what is a PFL-style meal on the go. Yes, it's possible to order strategically at most places when dining out and on the go. After all, you want to really enjoy your chance to eat outside your typical way of life. Make it count by planning and knowing your strategy well enough to incorporate it with unexpected food outings.

Conclusion: Enjoy It!

You're not hurting yourself by having an indulgence meal, so be sure to enjoy it. Incorporate your favorite foods—there is no food you are ever saying goodbye to forever. I definitely look forward to having my maple donuts, peanut butter and jelly sandwiches, Reese's Pieces with popcorn, and whole grain pancakes swimming in syrup with bacon and full eggs and cheese! Disciplined eating the majority of the time makes our favorite indulgence meals taste even more incredible than ever!

Indulgences are earned, not deserved, and are to be respected.

14

Triple S:

Sweeteners, Seasoning & Sauces

t's usually 2–3 weeks into the PFL method of eating that I get an email or text message from a client. It doesn't matter how many times I hear words like this, I smile and get excited for that person. Their message usually reads something like this:

I feel like I'm finally TASTING food! I never realized how unsatisfied my body was when I was putting the wrong things in it. Now I feel like I don't need to put much on my food because it tastes amazing! Thank you for teaching me how to re-train my body!

The only way you're going to stick to your new, healthy lifestyle is by making your food taste good. Food should be delicious, or you won't stick to eating the things you should. I giggle over all of the social media memes and jokes that rail on "dieting" because it is so bland and is so tasteless. Well, these people who still think this way need to try the PFL way! You deserve to eat delicious food every day. It's possible to eat delicious and savory meals that satisfy you and your cravings without packing excess grease, sugar, and harmful chemicals into your body.

It's even interesting to analyze the food intake of people who believe they are eating healthfully when their food is, in fact, drowning in sauces and sweeteners. Both of these can throw off the energy and chemical balance of your body, and turn a healthy meal into a fat-burn sabotage meal. I love helping to clean up a person's intake so they can see faster results in less time. Even small changes go a long way in providing the fat-burning, nutrient-absorbing environment we are trying to create in your body.

Why Processed Foods are So Delicious

You've probably grown so accustomed to eating factory-processed foods that your taste buds' ability to recognize true flavor has been diminished. Because of these artificial presences, many processed foods give your body just a taste of something so blissful that you continue to want more. Let's be honest, the food industry doesn't care about your health; they care about their profit margins. Food and food-like products is a business and you're the consumer—so it's time to become an informed consumer.

I'd like to give you several insights into the food industry and what they're doing to get you to eat their food, which naturally increases their bottom line:

• Highly-processed foods may have fiber and nutrients decreased, if not removed altogether. These components are largely responsible for slowing digestion and signaling feelings of satisfaction and being full. If you're not getting that natural stimulus because they've been reduced or removed, you will continue to eat past normal fullness—this is called overeating.

• Many foods have been chemically altered in taste tests. The food scientists tweak the tastes to be the epitome of perfection to stimulate the release of dopamine in your brain when you eat that food. Dopamine is the pleasure neurotransmitter which plays a large role in addiction. When you obtain happiness or other pleasurable feelings from eating food, of course you will want to continue eating, and you will turn to that food often for that sensation.

It's even worse because you won't feel satisfied very easily—it's scientifically difficult to achieve because of how these products are chemically structured. Normal triggers for your hormones to signal satiety aren't there. This is how you can go through an entire pint of ice cream or tray of Oreos™ without blinking an eye—your stomach's signals of being full are completely overridden by your taste buds' desire for more. I will always remember the day I learned about how Doritos® chips go through a series of obtaining the perfect taste. I finally knew why I could plow through an entire bag without it phasing me! I am now a much wiser consumer. Doritos® still taste amazing to me, but I know the secret weapon so I can keep myself from becoming a victim of ignorance. Though Doritos® is just the example I am using, this applies to so many food items in your grocery store.

• High Fructose Corn Syrup (HFCS), sugar, and Monosodium Glutamate (MSG) have all been linked to weight gain and obesity. They all enhance the flavor of the foods you eat and, let's face it, they make foods taste delicious! As you start looking at the ingredient labels on foods you regularly consume, you may be surprised to see these ingredients appearing in many foods you love. I was flabbergasted when I started becoming more aware and making an effort to get these particular additives out of the foods I eat. As a woman who has not yet had children, I especially find it interesting to learn the correlation between excessive fructose intake and adverse metabolic effects in the children of mothers who consumed HFCS and higher sugar amounts during pregnancy. Many studies have found an increased addiction and propensity to sugar in the children of these mothers. This knowledge led me to write the supplement to *The Power Foods Lifestyle, Power Foods for Two: a Healthy Lifestyle for the Pregnant Woman*. This booklet is available on www.body-buddies.com.

• The oils used in most processed foods are refined, meaning they are stripped of essential fatty acids that are necessary for healthy blood sugar levels, memory, and moods. As you regularly consume these types of foods in place of natural, wholesome foods with healthy oils, your heart, hormones, and brain may all be adversely impacted. Trans fats in many oils are also the number-one cause of high cholesterol in many people. I hope you are not terribly frustrated with me as you start to read your labels and find just how much soybean oil, vegetable oil, cottonseed oil, canola oil, and corn oil is in the foods you eat. I agree it is frustrating to learn that foods you love are slowly depriving you of your health. I hope, instead, you get frustrated with the food companies and take initiative to teach others what you are learning so we all become more informed consumers. If consumers stop buying these types of products and begin voicing their concerns, sooner or later, companies will have to listen and change.

• Processed foods employ many chemicals that don't naturally occur in foods. This includes additives and preservatives that help food last longer without going rancid. These foods are made for a long shelf life, not for long human life. Their packaging is strategic. The words and slogans they use are designed to emotionally entice you to buy their product—and the taste is intended to lock you in as customer for life. The more often you put these foods in your body, the more often you are not getting naturally-occurring vitamins and minerals which aid your body in everyday processes. Over time, deficiencies in these micronutrients will manifest themselves in small things like hair loss, bruising, circle under the eyes, weak bones, brittle nails, or more life-threatening illness and disease.

It's time to re-train your mind and your body to taste food differently. You will do this by following the instructions in this chapter on how to utilize sweeteners, sauces, and seasonings to not only amplify your power foods' natural flavors, but to train your mind to actually enjoy the natural flavors the food has to offer. My suggestions are a simple compilation of what I use on a day-to-day basis and have recommended for hundreds of people over the past few years. Please do your research and don't be afraid to try something that is not listed below.

Sweeteners

Oh that sweet, yummy taste that we all love! It triggers our pleasure centers and provides us with comfort, happiness, and temporary relief from stress. It's okay to like sweet food, but let's start looking for better ways to achieve a natural sweetness, rather than a chemically-pumped and enhanced sweetness that is over the top and quite addicting.

As you seek to learn the best options for yourself and your body, please keep in mind that I don't want you to go overboard and become a weirdo about food. I'm serious. There's no need to isolate yourself from people or events that will provide foods to you that I'm teaching you to avoid. Likewise, please don't feel badly if it takes you some time to change. Take baby steps in improving the foods you eat—this is not an all-or-nothing event! It's such a process, and I urge you to be patient! Take your own speed, and simply seek to make progress as you become more informed and aware of what you put in your body.

Honey is more than just sugar, it has over a hundred different compounds of minerals, amino acids, and vitamins but only if it is pure honey. A study conducted at Texas A&M University found that nearly 76% of the honey sampled from grocery store chains and drugstores had all the pollen removed. Fast food honey was also found to have 100% of the pollen removed. In order to gain the health benefits from honey, you need the pollen. Purchasing your honey at farmers' markets or natural products stores will pretty much guarantee you are purchasing the real deal.

With this recommendation, please don't think that honey doesn't impact your blood sugar levels. It does. It is processed just like sugar. However, if you really need your foods sweetened, this is the healthiest and most natural of options. When striving for ultimate fat loss, I encourage you to cut sweeteners out altogether, or use Stevia which I'll talk about a bit later on. You will find in the collection of Power Foods Recipe Books that honey is the main sweetener I use in recipes that call for a sweetener. Only rarely do I employ the use of other sweeteners, and when I do, it is for the sake of a "better alternative" than the regularly-consumed food item you may be eating. I haven't had white sugar or flour in my home for the past three years. While it's up to you if you cut this (it's not to say you don't eat it on indulgence meals), I found that by keeping it out of my house, I used wise substitutes in my baked goods way more often than using something "simple and easy" out of habit.

Many people use Agave Nectar, believing it's a healthy sweetener to use. This is a vegan alternative to honey. According to the American Journal of Clinical Nutrition, Agave has about five times lower impact on blood sugar than table sugar. The Agave plant grows natively in the southern United States and Mexico and has been used for hundreds of years in native Mexican culture for medicinal and sweetening purposes. However, due to the refining and processing of this plant to produce the product you see on your grocery store shelves, there are many controversial studies on this sweetener.

The debate often turns to Agave having a very high fructose content (simple sugar), which an overabundance of fructose has been shown to cause metabolic damage and raise triglycerides in the blood. I personally do not use the product. I like honey, and use it as a part of a healthy lifestyle when I need something sweet. If you choose to use Agave nectar, please look for a USDA-certified organic product or Quality Assurance International (QAI) certified-organic stamp.

Note: Please keep in mind that if you are pushing your body to lower-than-average body fat levels like many of the fitness competitors I train, even natural products like honey should be avoided as you should avoid any spike in blood sugar that is not strategically planned to benefit your aesthetic goals.

Artificial Sweeteners

Surely you have heard by now that artificial sweeteners are not all they appear to be. They can seem like a great alternative for those on a restricted caloric intake due to their "calorie-free" claims. That lovely phrase of "sugar-free" can cause choruses of praise to sing in your head!

However, be warned— just because a product claims there is no sugar, there surely is a chemical alternative to get your food or drink to taste good. No matter what you put in your mouth, there will be a chemical consequence in your body, good or bad. It's important that you set your own standards of what you will allow in your body, then always honor that.

The Harvard School of Public Health teaches that diet soda can be a short-term substitute for adults weaning themselves off sugary soda, but cautions for kids to avoid artificial sweeteners in beverages altogether as the long-term effects are still unknown.[12]

Here are some interesting statements on these sweeteners that may help you begin forming your own guidelines:

• Our bodies don't excrete 100% of artificial sweeteners, so something remains in the body. Chemicals like these may impact your hormones, which are equally responsible for the fat loss environment, along with portion control and nutrient pairing you put in your body.

• Just because a food product claims "no sugar" doesn't mean it's totally truthful! The Food and Drug Administration allows nutrition labels to claim zero calories if there are five or less calories per serving of a food.

• While artificial sweeteners may be derived from a natural source, the extraction and processing methods are so extensive that the sweetener no longer resembles what nature once provided. Their chemical structures have been changed. Is there any wonder that you feel bloated, constipated, or fatigued while regularly consuming artificial sweeteners? If you were to eliminate all artificial sweeteners (including drinks, gums, pre-workouts, etc.), there's no doubt you will feel much more alive, energetic, and lack the dreaded bloat.

• The human brain responds to sweetness by signaling you to eat more. When you have an artificially-sweetened product or beverage and provide the sweet taste without any calories, you can actually crave more sweet foods and drinks. This can easily lead to you eating excess calories.

• Be aware that most protein powders, pre-workouts, and Branched-Chain Amino Acid powders utilize artificial sweeteners like Sucralose in order to keep their carbohydrate content lower. If one of my clients exhibits sensitivities toward Sucralose, we usually find that using an egg-based protein, Stevia-sweetened protein powder (like IsoNatural), or skipping a protein shake all together helps immensely. With these clients, I usually design their own "stack" for a pre-workout (combination of supplements and vitamins in pill form) in order to get the sucralose out of their body. Not all individuals need a pre-workout stack—only those training for specific performance or aesthetic goals.

---

[12] http://www.hsph.harvard.edu/nutritionsource/healthy-drinks/artificial-sweeteners/

• If you feel you need your foods to be sweet all the time, you might consider pulling back from natural and artificial sweeteners altogether. I like to use this analogy in helping us understand they're actually hiding the natural taste of foods. Instead of masking the taste, try to enhance their natural characteristics and flavors.

Stevia: This is a plant naturally grown in Brazil and Paraguay that is sweeter than sugar—about 250-300 times sweeter! Due to its high sweetness factor, use of the extract requires about 1/5 the amount of table sugar. Extraction of the stevia leaf includes crushing the leaf, extracting the water, filtering and separating the liquid from plant material, purifying the extract with water or food grade alcohol, and drying. More than 5,000 food and beverage products use Stevia throughout the world. There are liquid drops of Stevia available that many people find works well for their use in foods and beverages. It also has the potential for lowering blood sugar levels, so diabetics should keep this in mind when using the sweetener.

Truvia™: Though the marketing is good at making you think so, Truvia is not an equivalent to Stevia. Stevia is not even listed in the first three ingredients on its label. Just like other artificial sweeteners (and yes, we are going to label this as artificial as it's chemically derived), your body doesn't know how to metabolize the chemical structures, which may interfere with your hormones and metabolism. This is very problematic for you when trying to lose body fat. Its main ingredient, Erythritol, is a sugar alcohol made by processing genetically modified corn. Sugar alcohols are known for their side effects of gastric distress, cramping, gas, and bloating. Sound like fun?

Sucralose: Also known as Splenda, sucralose is one of the most frequently-used artificial sweeteners in beverages and foods to make these products sugar-free. Let's take a look at the chemistry behind sucralose: it starts off as a sugar molecule (a disaccharide that contains glucose and fructose), but then in the factory, three chlorine molecules are added to this structure which makes it a foreign object to our bodies. While this sweetener doesn't seem to impact insulin, making it the best option for Type I and Type II Diabetes populations, sucralose is still under scrutiny for any potential links to diseases or disorders. I will not, and I repeat, will not be surprised when evidence is revealed in the next 10-20 years that sucralose is, in fact, linked to disorders that we see on the rise in the United States.[13]

Aspartame: This sweetener that is found mostly in Diet Coke® and over 9,000 other products in the United States is actually 10% methanol—a poison. Aspartame has long been the focus of many activists to get off the shelves of our grocery stores as tests conducted on lab rats have found that the chemical may have a role in causing cancer.

Now, remember we need to take all studies with a grain of salt and look at the control factors. In each of the studies I have read, the dosage used on the rats was far beyond the dosage a human consumer might get by drinking a 12 oz. can of Diet Coke®.

I don't provide that information to indicate that Aspartame, or any artificial sweetener for that matter, is okay to be ingesting. I hope you are past the point of asking, "Can I have it?" and are now asking "Why should, or shouldn't I choose to have it? How can I moderately use this?"

There are other sweeteners, and will continue to be others, that pop up and are marketed to you with deceptive appeal. You may or may not be lured into believing clever slogans and marketing tactics.

Bring it Home

Do yourself a favor and take an inventory of all the artificial sweeteners you are currently putting in your body—including salad dressing, gum, soda, protein powders, pre-workout supplements, BCAAs, and flavored water beverages. You might be surprised to see just how many are a part of your normal habits. In order to help your body function more efficiently and decrease the chances of illness or disease, see if you can't work to eliminate one of your regularly-used sweeteners each week.

A car with a beautiful exterior is only as valuable as how it runs under the hood. Likewise, a healthy and fit-looking body on the outside is only as good as its health on the inside. Be wise in your use of artificial sweeteners if you can't eliminate them all together.

Sauces

Sauces can easily take a well-balanced meal and turn it into a fat-storage-promoting meal. I will admit I love the taste of barbeque sauce as much as the next person, but I realize that the high carbohydrate, fat and sugar ratio will cause my blood sugar to be impacted—especially if I'm eating a PVF meal where I'm trying to minimize any impact on blood sugar. Choose to use sauces that don't have more than

---

[13] All of the information discussed in this book is to increase your awareness, and provide you with enough information to formulate your personal standard of how to treat your body. There is hardly any "non-strategic" item I discuss in this book that I have cut from my life for the long haul. Instead, I employ, and hope to see you employ as well, a mindset where those types of non-strategic foods that display evidence of potential harm are used in moderation as indulgences, not as a regular way of life.

the benchmark of 5–10 grams of sugar in everyday meals. Be sure to check for High Fructose Corn Syrup (HFCS) in every food item and sauce you purchase! HFCS is an industrial food product and doesn't occur naturally within substances. This means that your body doesn't know how to handle it. The molecular ratio of glucose and fructose bound together in an unnatural form causes many digestive and metabolic issues that, in short, lead to over-consumption of total calories.

Below are some great ways to dress up your food with select types of sauces. Following PFL principles should not be boring or bland. Seek to enjoy your food! This will happen as you really pay attention to the next section on spices as well.

Ranch Dressing: Make your own Ranch dressing using my recipe in Volume I of the Power Foods Lifestyle Recipe books, or use the powdered form to sprinkle on a salad topped with cottage cheese. Bolthouse Farms® also makes an incredible line of yogurt-based dressings that taste delicious and are all within PFL guidelines. I use their Ranch dressing a lot!

Mustards: Dijon, Brown, Regular—they all offer so much flavor! It's amazing how many foods taste great with mustard on them. Be brave and try something new. I especially love mixing a bit of Dijon in a can of tuna.

Italian Dressing: A little bit can go a long way. Marinade your chicken in this, or dress your salads with it (lightly, of course). Avoid the fat-free or light varieties as they use artificial sweeteners and additives to make up for the chemical change; simply use smaller amounts of the full-fat versions as this is better for your body's digestion.

Ketchup: Used in moderation (about 1 Tbsp. per serving), this is a sauce that can dress up many foods. I like to use ketchup with my egg whites and complex carb mixes (like lentils, black beans, and brown rice). Be aware there is some sugar in this product, so go light and use an organic product. You can even make your own using my recipe in Volume I of the Power Foods Lifestyle Recipe Books.

Soy Sauce: This Asian deliciousness has a bad reputation due to its outrageous sodium content, but it can add much variety and flavor to your meats and vegetables when you use it lightly. However, if you have high blood pressure and your doctor has asked you to avoid sodium, this should be a sauce to avoid. Whether or not you have high blood pressure, seek to use a low-sodium sauce. Most Asian diners will provide this to you upon request.

Salsa & Hot Sauce: This is one of the best toppings you can use for salads, meats, potatoes, veggies, and egg whites as there is a lot of flavor packed into one serving. Be sure to double-check the sugar content and remember our principle of watching out for foods over the 5-10 grams of sugar mark. Salsa is a definite must-have for your refrigerator.

BBQ/Teriyaki Sauces: The biggest culprit in these sauces is the high carbohydrate to sugar ratio. If you can find a sauce that has less than 5 grams of either of these items on the food label (without the product using artificial sweeteners as a substitute to reach these lower numbers) then feel free to use these types of sauces in moderation. I have found that a good Mesquite BBQ seasoning can come pretty close to producing the same taste as a normal BBQ sauce. Watch out for HFCS in these sauces!

Seasonings

Nothing makes me feel more like a gourmet chef than opening my cupboard and choosing a random assortment of spices and herbs to add to my meals. As you follow PFL principles, you may use natural seasonings in combinations that are endless—the sky's the limit! I have many clients who are initially hesitant in trying new combinations, but once they begin experimenting, they realize how much fun it is. Realizing how capable they are of making any basic meal into a mouthwatering masterpiece is a great part of their lifestyle change! As you try the PFL recipes I have created, you will learn that you don't need a ton of seasonings to make food flavors POP and taste delicious!

If you're someone who doesn't have many seasonings or spices in your home, let's fix that. Head over to find Amazon on your Internet browser and type into the search bar the phrase "small glass spice jars." You can find some very inexpensive sets. Purchase 1 or 2 sets, then go to your local store that carries these items in bulk to purchase the dry ingredients. It is much less expensive than purchasing an herb or spice rack that is already made for you.

Also keep in mind that you don't need to drop a ton of money at once to do this. Take everything in stride. Perhaps one week you purchase the jars. Then each consecutive week you can purchase 1-2 new seasonings or herbs. Make this an enjoyable process of improvement, rather than a sudden dent in your wallet over which you later become frustrated.

Be sure that your cupboard is stocked with some of the basics I have listed below and use frequently in the PFL Recipe Books:

- Basil
- Bay Leaves
- Cajun Seasonings
- Celery Salt
- Chicken Bouillon (non-SG)
- Chili Powder
- Cinnamon Cumin
- Coconut flavoring
- Coriander
- Curry Powder
- Garlic Powder
- Garlic Salt
- Italian Seasoning
- Lemon Pepper
- Mesquite BBQ
- Nutmeg
- Onion Powder
- Oregano
- Parsley Flakes
- Red Pepper Flakes
- Rosemary
- Sea Salt (or pink Himalayan salt)
- Seasoned Salt (non-MSG)
- Thai Green Paste
- Thyme
- Turmeric
- Vanilla

Let's get started with a few different combinations to try. These are great because they work with many foods from chicken and fish to vegetables and soups. You will learn to love the taste of real home-cooked food!

Southwestern Seasoning Blend

2 1/2 Tbsp. Chili Powder

1 Tbsp. Coriander

1 Tbsp. Sea Salt

1 Tbsp. Oregano

2 Tbsp. Paprika

1 tsp. Pepper

2 tsp. Cumin

1 tsp. Cayenne Pepper

Sweet and Zesty Spice

2 Tbsp. Cinnamon

1 1/2 tsp. Ginger

1 1/2 tsp. Nutmeg

Taco Seasoning

1 Tbsp. Chili Powder

2 tsp. Onion Powder

1 tsp. Cumin

1 tsp. Garlic Powder

1 tsp. Paprika

1 tsp. Oregano

1 tsp. Sugar

1/2 tsp. Sea Salt

Now here's what you've been waiting for . . . my secret blends! I put these on nearly everything I make. If you are someone who has high blood pressure and has been counseled by your doctor to watch your sodium intake, then it would be wise to cut any salt measurements in half. However, if this is not something you need to worry about, you will be just fine adding salts to your food. Sodium intake only becomes a problem when we are eating so many processed foods that use sodium in extraordinary amounts as a preservative to increase shelf life. If you are getting in a good workout where you are sweating and eating Power Foods, please add salt to your meals! Your body needs this wonderful electrolyte to maintain balance on the intracellular level.

Kristy's Secret Blend #1

1 Tbsp. Garlic Salt

1 tsp. Cinnamon

2 tsp. Oregano

Kristy's Secret Blend #2

2 tsp. Curry Powder

1 tsp. Turmeric

3 Chicken Bouillon Cubes (mashed)

1 tsp. Garlic Salt

1/2 tsp. Chili Powder

Kristy's Secret Blend #3

1 Tbsp. Garlic Salt

2 tsp. Italian Seasoning

1 tsp. Onion Powder

2 tsp. Cajun Seasoning

1 tsp. Red Pepper Flakes

1/2 tsp. Celery Salt

Conclusion

Learn to love the natural tastes of food. Relish them. Savor them. Learn to season your food and become the master label reader in your family and workplace. A small amount of knowledge can go a long way as you seek to apply the principles you are learning about traps and tricks the food industry uses—become the master of yourself by using a new strategy in how you eat. The PFL strategy will help your body find a healthy state of function where you feel incredible and in control.

15

Supplements & Vitamins

N o supplement has the power to benefit your body above what balanced and nutritious eating habits and exercise can do. If there is one thing that bothers me more than car salespeople, it's supplements salespeople. This is because they will promise you results to get you to purchase the product. This doesn't mean that the products are bad, per sé. This simply means that we should not be using supplements to get results for which we are not willing to first adjust in our eating and exercise behavior.

I can't tell you how often I have stood in a gym supplement shop to purchase particular products I use and listened to the completely flawed information that was used to sell an individual on a product. I am careful in these situations not to overstep my bounds and come across as the know-it-all-sales-stealer, but when the situation is right, I do open my mouth.

One particular situation involved a fat burner (that included a banned substance) and a very overweight woman who was asking the young man behind the counter if it would help her shed her weight. After letting my "BS radar" go off for enough time, I kindly stepped in and asked if I might provide a little education on the product so she could be a more informed consumer. After the customer left with my card and no fat burner, I apologized to the salesman, who actually thanked me. "I didn't know that," he said, referring to the information I had provided to the two of them. "I'm glad you said something. I don't want to sell a bad product." I then spoke with him for the next fifteen minutes to give him an overview of particular products that would be better for that particular demographic of people. I even went so far as to tell him just how important his position was. "You're like a pharmacist without a license," I said, "with a great potential to mess a person's body up. Treat your job with great importance." I challenged him to study the products he would be selling so he could best recommend them. He accepted my challenge.

The meaning of the word supplements is *in addition to*, yet those marketing these pills and concoctions aren't the ones to teach you what you should be doing with your nutrition. After all, money isn't made by telling people to eat their vegetables, it's made by selling products.

When used correctly, supplements can be wonderful. But until you are cleaning up your eating habits, you cannot expect a pill or powder to do the work for you. They are not a replacement or the sole cause of results. I don't care which celebrities are telling you that a particular product or supplement changed their life—they don't tell you all of the other things they were doing which also contributed to their success. You need to understand that people are paid to endorse products.

The goal of many fitness competitors is to attain a sponsorship from a supplement company to offset the cost of their competition training expenses. Once attained, the fitness competitor is "married" to the company and has strict requirements of social media posts and other endorsements in order to keep the sponsorship. In other words, these people are promoting a product to you for their profit—not yours. Now please keep in mind that I do know several individuals and companies who do a good job of upholding integrity in this supplement industry. They go to great lengths to promote products they believe in and have used prior to the sponsorship, and I applaud them for their integrity!

Please open your eyes and look at the business behind products so you are not emotionally manipulated into purchasing something that will leave you frustrated and disappointed.

#1 Misused Supplement

Let's revisit that situation with the woman and the fat burner, as I'm sure you felt cheated—you wanted to know why I felt strongly enough to say something, right?

At the age of 19, fat burners (thermogenics) became a part of my life. Though already fit, my goal was to lose more weight and attain a very lean and sculpted physique. I was a college student who was spending six hours per day in dance rehearsals. I carried the bottle of fat burners in my purse and took one with every meal, before rehearsal, and before my workouts. I can still taste the unique burn in my mouth and throat as I think about those years. Terror engulfed me whenever I ran low on my supply, and I quickly ordered a new bottle. In my mind, the fat burners were the only reason I was as lean as I was, especially with my binge-eating struggles.

These supplements make great claims—the agents in fat burners *do* have metabolism-boosting components which stimulate thermogenesis and enable enzymes in your body to break down and transport food to your cells more quickly. These components also provide energy because they contain exorbitant amounts of caffeine. The typical dosage of 2–3 pills daily contain anywhere from 100-250 milligrams of caffeine. Caffeine is a natural fat-burning agent, so nearly all supplements contain very high dosages. However, caffeine is a stimulant and can quickly lose its effect as your body adapts to it.

While fat burners have metabolic-enhancing agents that make it feasible to market them as such, here is the simple fact you must understand: fat burners do not expel fat from the body. Instead, they may help your body burn more fat by first, stimulating your body to process more quickly and be more energetic for a brief period of time (3-4 hours), thus, burning more calories than you otherwise might. This increase in energy enables you to be more active all around. There is no magic to them—just a simple pattern of cause and effect. Fat burners may also help suppress your appetite so you aren't as likely to eat as much.

Their name is genius, as who doesn't want to burn fat? They're glamorized and over-sold to the masses for this emotional pull without any additional information for consumers. However, without a nutritious and strategic eating method dedicated to laying the foundation for the fat burners to be strategic, there is no point to using them. The one exception includes fitness competitors or models who are "dialing in" to that utmost shredded point of leanness. These are people who have their nutrition and training dialed in to a tee, with zero wavering in the face of tempting sweets and foods exempt from their meal plans. When all variables are in perfect control as such, fat burners can be the extra edge in the final 3-4 weeks prior to competition. However, be warned, my friends who fit in this description, that once you start eating larger portions and neglecting your reverse diet protocol, your body will be at a higher propensity to store fat. Always consider if the risk is worth the reward, and become the master of yourself through education and discipline.

This next discussion point applies not only to fat burners, but pre-workouts, and other caffeine or energy products. Because your body can quickly develop a high tolerance for stimulants, you may think you need more in order to feel them working. This may lead to an overdose and damaged organs, including your liver and kidneys. Fat burners, as with any supplement containing caffeine, are something that must be correctly rotated with a few weeks on and a few weeks off. Without this cycling effect, caffeine-infused supplements can completely disengage the abilities of the adrenal glands (located on top of the kidneys) and later cause issues with the thyroid. Adrenal Fatigue Syndrome impacts many people in the United States without their even being aware of it. Symptoms of AFS include feeling tired for no reason, difficulty bouncing back from stress or illness, feeling rundown and overwhelmed, and having difficulty getting up in the morning, even when going to bed at a reasonable hour.

Take care not to trust just anyone's advice when it comes to supplements—even mine! Learn to do your own research and know what you're putting in your body. I have seen far too many people take something that should never have been recommended for their current condition and goals, and wonder why their body was responding so poorly (rapid heartbeat, flushing, swelling, etc.). Learn to shop online where you can read as much information about a product (both pros and cons), and purchase with your own free will instead of being "suckered" into a purchase by a slick salesperson.

At the end of this chapter, I have included a general overview of vitamins and supplements I feel are appropriate for the general population and have regularly recommended for clients over the past few years. Am I a doctor? Nope, we have already established that. So use this information as a springboard to doing your own research in order to make a wise decision for yourself. Exceptions always apply to every statement I make.

Let's Not Forget About Vitamins

Vitamin deficiencies happen when you don't get enough of a certain vitamin in your food intake. Deficiencies can increase your risk for health problems including heart disease, cancer, and osteoporosis. Once again, *blah, blah, blah*, right? We know that we need to get our vitamins and minerals, but the question is how do we do this regularly? And the question I hear most often is this: *Can't I just take a pill that will take care of it all?*

Living by the PFL will help you get nearly all of the daily vitamins your body needs. However, if you have specific health problems, it's important to consult with your physician about the proper intake amounts of supplements and vitamins. In addition, if you have a particular nutritional need, I highly recommend scheduling a consultation with one of the Body Buddies coaches as they can tailor the PFL strategies and foods to best fit your needs.

There are 13 essential vitamins needed in the body in order for your cells to *function*, grow, and develop normally:

1. Vitamin A
2. Vitamin C
3. Vitamin D
4. Vitamin E
5. Vitamin K

6. Vitamin B1 (Thiamine)

7. Vitamin B2 (Riboflavin)

8. Vitamin B3 (Niacin)

9. Pantothenic Acid

10. Biotin

11. Vitamin B6

12. Vitamin B12

13. Folate (folic acid)

One way you can see your current levels of your vitamin intake is to choose one day each week and enter your daily meals into a tracker like MyFitnessPal, FitBit, or CalorieCount. There are many applications you can download for free, or minimal charge on your smart phone that will work for this task. After entering your daily meals, check the report on vitamins and see where your levels fall. After doing this enough times, you will begin to see a pattern for which vitamins you're easily satisfying the recommendations, and which vitamins you need to consider supplementing. Though I do not encourage regular daily food logging, it can be helpful when trying to determine whether or not your meals are meeting your needs.

General Overview

Below is a list of supplements and vitamins that you may want to consider in conjunction with your strategic eating method. I am a true believer in obtaining as many nutrients as possible from real food. However, there most certainly can be a time and a place for these additions. When used strategically, the items in this list can be beneficial to you as you work to improve your health. I could write an entire chapter on each one of the items in this list; however, I'm going to keep it simple, and allow you to do your own research to explore further. A consultation with a Body Buddies coach can help you choose which of the list below will be most beneficial for you to implement in your lifestyle.

Be sure to check out the Products page at www.body-buddies.com to see some of the products I use and recommend.

Protein Powder: While definitely not a "must," this is very helpful for convenience and speed's sake. Protein helps muscles to repair and rebuild, especially when making a change in your body composition (body fat to lean muscle tissue) is your end goal.

There are many forms of protein powder that can aid you in your goals to get adequate amounts of protein in your daily intake. Incorporating protein powder into 1–2 of your meals each day enables you to get a higher amount of protein intake without consuming purely animal proteins. With that said, I don't recommend more than two servings of protein powder per day. Try to get your other meals from whole food sources.

1. **Whey Protein:** One of the two major components in milk, whey contains our macronutrients of protein, fats, and carbohydrates as well as vitamins and minerals. It is one of the fastest-digesting proteins available so it absorbs into your body immediately. Your body will not absorb the full amount of protein in whey, so keep that in mind with the balancing of your numbers. I don't believe it's necessary to become so obsessed with perfection in numbers that we manipulate every little thing we do for maximum results; however, it is an interesting fact to be aware of.

• *Whey Concentrate:* Whey concentrate is created by pushing the liquid portion of milk through a filter. During this process, material that is left behind is dried and forms whey concentrate. This form of protein must be broken down by your body into the amino acids that construct the three-dimensional structure. Concentrate is usually higher in carbohydrates than isolates. Whey contains only trace elements of lactose, the natural sugar found in milk. This makes whey possible to digest for most people, but the exceptions are always out there. Whey concentrate is less processed than whey isolates.

• *Whey Isolates:* Isolates are simply pure protein with very little of dairy elements leftover. During this process, the original three-dimensional structure of the proteins are denatured, or broken down, into its amino acid building blocks. This denaturing is the same process that happens in your body, but as isolates are already broken down, this type of protein can be absorbed very rapidly into your system. This makes isolates the most ideal post-workout protein. It releases amino acids which rush to aid your muscles after working to break them down. Whey Isolates are a higher-priced item, but that is due to isolate containing more protein than casein at 90-94% protein. Be careful not to use an isolate for a meal replacement as you'll find it won't keep you full for long as it absorbs and is utilized by your body so quickly.

o The Power Foods Lifestyle recipes containing protein powder are made using Whey Isolate powders in order to manipulate and strategize the carbohydrate count for the meal. When making these recipes with a concentrate, you'll need to account for anywhere from 5-15 additional carbs per serving in the recipe.

• *Whey Hydrolysate:* An expensive pre-digested whey protein, whey hydrolysate is heavily marketed as a trendy item. Though virtually free of potential allergens, I have yet to find studies that clearly indicate a boost in the bioavailability of the product above that of a whey concentrate or isolate powder.

2. *Casein Protein*: This is a slow-digesting protein derived from cow's milk that helps keep you feeling fuller longer. Due to this, casein is perfect for a meal replacement or pre-bedtime snack. It supplies a steady influx of amino acids to help retain muscle mass, meaning this is great not only for those looking to build lean muscle tissue, but also elderly people as well as busy people who don't have time to eat much.

3. *Soy Protein:* Soy protein often gets a bad rap as some studies suggest that the phytoestrogens found in soy protein can increase estrogen levels and decrease testosterone. However, phytoestrogens also contribute to lowered risk of osteoporosis, heart disease, and breast cancer. Soy is neither the good guy, nor the bad guy. It can be a great alternative for you if you're lactose intolerant or sensitive to whey.

4. *Plant Protein:* High-quality plant proteins are great for Vegans, Vegetarians, or those who are lactose-intolerant. The three main types of plant protein are hemp, pea, and brown rice. In my opinion, these proteins do not taste as good as other sources of protein, but provide an extremely healthy and clear-cut way to get your protein. Be aware that the carbohydrate content can often be higher in plant protein than a whey isolate.

5. *Egg Protein:* This protein is extremely bio-available and delivers very high protein quality. Egg protein is naturally dairy-free and so a good alternative for those who experience lactose intolerance or milk allergies.

Pre-workout: Prime your body for your workout by providing the amino acids and vitamins that will help it best respond to intense exercise. Those who are not engaging in over 30 minutes of intense resistance training should not need a pre-workout. If it's caffeine alone you need for energy, go with a straight caffeine tablet and spare your body the additional amino acids that aren't needed.

Choose a pre-workout drink with no more than 100-200 mg caffeine (most will fall in this range) per serving. Never consume more than this for a pre-workout as it can really cause you to crash afterward and potentially lead to heart problems. Most pre-workouts contain L-Glutamine (aids in repairing muscle damage), Beta Alanine (responsible for the itchiness), Nitric Oxide (regulates blood flow and interacts with almost every protein), and Taurine (an antioxidant-like amino acid that protects your cells from damage), which all aid your muscle recovery and ability to push harder in your workout.

Take your pre-workout drink or stack 30 minutes before your workout begins so your body has time to absorb the caffeine and begin to utilize it. If you are a natural athlete (meaning you don't use banned substances, anabolic agents, test boosters, etc.), read your labels and do not drink anything with Geranium or 1, 3 Dimethylamalamine (DMAA) as these are on the banned substances list. In combination with caffeine, these stimulants can cause cardiovascular problems like heart attacks. Although 1, 3 DMAA was banned by the Food and Drug Administration in 2012, many companies have continued to distribute pre-workouts, fat burners, and other supplements still containing these dangerous chemicals. Until we can be sure this chemical is entirely out of products on the shelves, learn to check your labels.

BCAAs (Branched-Chain Amino Acids): BCAAs aid protein synthesis and enhance your workout, making them a very effective supplement for those wishing to develop more lean muscle tissue. Amino acids are the "building blocks" of proteins. When you don't get enough of even one of the nine essential amino acids (branched-chain amino acids are included in the nine), your body's proteins begin to break down. Make sure the ratio of leucine to isoleucine and valine is 2:1:1 by checking the back of the label. Many companies utilize a higher leucine ratio, but studies have found this does not make a great difference. Drink one serving of BCAAs starting 30 minutes prior to your workout and throughout the workout (intraworkout). You can do this by getting a quarter gallon water bottle or jug and filling it with water to drink during that time. Have another serving of BCAAs at the opposite time of day as your workout. If training in the morning, that means do another serving in the evening.

L-Glutamine: This is a naturally-occurring amino acid in your body that is the most plentiful of all amino acids. You will need to supplement this amino acid when putting your body through the extra physical stress that is required to change your body composition. For muscle toning and growth, consume L-glutamine in the morning on an empty stomach, 30 minutes pre-workout, and if chasing muscle gains earnestly, at night before sleeping. Do not heat glutamine as it will destroy its helpful properties. It is best absorbed in powder form. Try mixing it with water or your protein shake.

Kre-Alkalyn/Creatine Monohydrate: Kre-Alkalyn is the newest and arguably best form of creatine, and the only creatine that has a U.S. Patent for stability and purity. Kre-Alkalyn's pH-Correct technology keeps you from bloating and cramping, unlike creatine-monohydrate. Providing your body with this supplement enables your muscles to have increased access to phosphate, therefore generating ATP—a muscle energy source. This helps you develop lean muscle. The dosage of Kre-Alkalyn will vary between men and women according to their goals. Creatine monohydrate may be used as well. My general rule of thumb is to recommend creatine monohydrate initially for muscle gains clients, with us switching to Kre-Alkalyn if I sense any hesitation or fear of the "bloat" that can often accompany creatine supplementation. Take care to study proper cycling guidelines for either.

Multi-Vitamin: Be sure to choose a high-quality vitamin so that your body absorbs as much of the vitamins as possible. Go to www.consumerlab.com to see if your brand of multi-vitamin has been found to contain all or more of what it claims. Most multi-vitamins have been found not to provide you with the full amounts they claim on their nutrition label. This is a large reason why you cannot rely on a pill to supply your body with all of the vital nutrients it needs to function well.

Iron: Be sure that you do not take this with your Calcium supplement—the two elements will cancel the other's properties and your body will not absorb anything. Iron is essential for muscle nourishment, as well as providing oxygen transportation by your blood supply. If you are not eating red meat at least once per week, iron should be a definite consideration to supplement.

Vitamin D-3: This vitamin plays a vital role in supporting your immune system as well as contributing to your neuromuscular function. D-3 also aids in the absorption of Calcium as well as boosts energy metabolism.

Calcium: This is a very important mineral for strength and bone development as you age. Women, especially, should pay heed to taking their daily recommended amount of

1,000 mg. Be sure to take Calcium with Vitamin D-3 to maximize absorption.

Magnesium Glycinate: This form of magnesium provides the highest levels of absorption and bioavailability. It plays a role in enzyme activity (which enables thousands of chemical processes in your body), but also plays a role in energy and ATP production (energy storage). Magnesium deficiencies play a far-reaching role in the breakdown of the body and boost brain function for both young and old. I can tell a very distinct difference in my moods when I take magnesium versus when I don't, which I have heard in similar statements from many clients as we have weekly coaching calls. This is an extremely important macro-mineral and my #1 most recommended vitamin for clients, above a multi-vitamin and fish oil.

B-Complex or Brewer's Yeast: B vitamins help your body convert food into glucose, which provides energy to your body. This complex is a group of vitamins that includes eight of the B vitamins, which play a variety of roles in your body. Brewer's Yeast is a complex with folic acid, B-12, Potassium, Thiamin, Niacin, and Chromium. It is a beneficial supplement for energy in all ages and genders, but especially for mothers who are breast-feeding as it naturally aids in milk production. I love hearing how clients feel after taking Brewer's Yeast.

CLA: Conjugated Linoleic Acid is a naturally occurring fatty acid that aids your metabolism and fat reduction efforts. Though it might sound counterproductive to many, its properties are such that when taken with your balanced-macros meals each day, it may contribute to lowering your body fat.

Fish Oil: These essential fatty acids (known as EFAs) are shown in many studies to serve as anti-inflammatory relief in your body, protein synthesis support for existing and new muscle tissue, and to support the brain and health as a person ages. Unless you are eating fish 4-5 times per week, fish oil supplementation is encouraged by many doctors and dietitians across the country, as well as the American Heart Association.

St. John's Wort: A natural remedy that boosts your mood and helps you not be so cranky and mean to your loved ones. This is especially good for ladies during that most glorious time of the month. Be sure that you do not utilize this herb if you are taking a prescription anti-depressant.

Conclusion

Be wise and do some research before putting any vitamin or supplement in your body, no matter who recommends you do so. Remember to take into consideration the absorbability of each item, as quality vs. cost is often evident in the good it will do in your body. A few quality items along with living the PFL principles are far more important and beneficial to your body than taking the full spectrum, but of lower grade and quality. Be sure to check out the incredible products at *nutrikey.net*. These products are pharmaceutical grade and regulated closely by dietitians.

16

Hydration

Isn't it miserable to want and need water, yet either not have any around, or be unable to have some (in the case of fasting for religious or civil purposes)? I think we all have experienced that at one time or another and it's awful! All that seems to matter in those times is finding and drinking water. The bodybuilding clients I work with often look at me with puppy-dog eyes and a sad face as they say, "all I want is water." (We utilize a process of dehydration to manipulate their body's appearance for judging for a time.) After all, water is the very foundation of all the physiological needs of your body.

So if you know how important water is to your body, why do you tend to not drink enough of it (unless you're already doing great at this principle!)? What is it about your daily life that keeps you from doing what you know is important?

This could be for many reasons. Our brains can only focus on so many things at once, and often, there are much greater stressors in the chaotic lives we live than drinking water. Time simply evades us and we get wrapped up in work, allowing many hours to pass without even a thought of hydration until thirst sets in. Many times, the natural consequence of an increased water intake (using the restroom more often), can be a great deterrent to our desire to hydrate ourselves effectively. Sometimes you just don't have time to get to the restroom every two hours, right? While these are valid reasons and surely what might be holding you back, I think the biggest factor is that you simply haven't made drinking water a daily habit.

There are many acts you do daily without a second thought. Every habit in your life is triggered by a stimulus of sight, smell, or sound; for instance, you may habitually wipe off your feet at the entryway upon entering your home each day. This action is triggered by the act of walking through the door, smelling the familiar scent of your home and seeing it the way you left it. It is a natural stimulus—one that you don't recognize until you begin analyzing your habits. You can use natural stimuli to trigger healthful habits. This is how you train yourself to have more beneficial behaviors that will improve your current and future life and body. *Be sure to listen to my podcast episode on Trigger Training—the Body Buddies Podcast may be found on iTunes or Stitcher Radio.*

It's time for you to make drinking water regularly a habit. It all will begin with a trigger that you train yourself to recognize. One of my triggers is seeing the jug of water that I carry with me everywhere I go. As I keep it on my desk while I work, on the front seat as I drive, and with me as I walk around the gym, I am reminded frequently to be guzzling it down.

As we go through this chapter, I would like you to begin thinking about how you can start triggering yourself to drink more water as well. One of the best triggers you can have is getting in the habit of waking up in the morning and immediately walking to the fridge and drinking two 8-ounce glasses of cold water. The trigger is waking up. The habit is drinking two cups of water. This action and reaction will produce a new habit that takes no effort in thought once in place. The result of this new habit is a happy body that is relieved from the water deficiency it experienced while you slept.

Water Intake Recommendation

My typical recommendation for average, healthy adults is as follows:

- Drink your body weight (lb.) in ounces of water or

- Drink approximately one gallon of water each day whichever seems more doable.

You may balk at this recommendation as the typical intake of people who I consult or lecture admit to an average daily intake of 40-50 oz. As I have stated many times prior to this, exceptions always apply. I have worked with elderly individuals who worked on drinking 60-70 ounces per day. I have worked with children and teenagers who also had a smaller requirement. Pregnant women additionally have a different recommendation, which I discuss in my book, *Power Foods for Two: A Lifestyle for the Pregnant Woman.* You should not be water-logging yourself. The take-away principle is to get in the habit of providing your body with the hydrating power it needs to work efficiently. With the exceptions stated, let's discuss the typical recommendation further.

Did you know there are 8 ounces in a cup and 128 ounces in a gallon? These are good measurements to memorize and remember from now on. Let's do some math together to determine how much water you should be drinking:

If you weigh 150 pounds and follow the recommendation of ounces per pound of body weight, you will be drinking 150 ounces of water. Take 150, divide it by 8, and we end up at 18.75 cups. As there are 16 cups in one gallon, you will be drinking just over a gallon of water. Perhaps this is too much for you and you are bloated and water-logged, so you might scale back and focus on the gallon mark. For most adults (who weigh over 128 lb.), the gallon of water is going to be the better approach to take.

This will probably be a lot more water in comparison to what you're currently drinking. While it seems difficult initially, take it in baby steps. Here are some tips to help you:

1. Stop sipping and start chugging. Every time you get a drink, take the lid off, open your throat, and get some real volume of water in your body. It's so easy to sip on water all day and think you are getting plenty of water when in actuality you aren't. As I always tell my clients: Pop the top and Chug-a-Lug!

2. Every time you get a drink of water, make the goal to swallow 8 times. It's amazing how much more you will drink than a simple 2-3 swallows. You'll surely accomplish your daily goal if you utilize this tip.

It may also help you to know there is a physiological need for true hydration in your body. When you consume more protein daily than normal (without increasing your water intake), your blood urea nitrogen level rises. Your kidneys are stressed a bit more by consuming more protein, so they produce more concentrated urine. Increasing your water intake helps your body function regularly. Your body naturally needs plenty of water to fuel bodily processes on all levels, so this is just an extra incentive to hydrate as you should. Your body is a complex machine of systems requiring water to work properly. Drinking enough water is the best thing you can do to aid your new healthy lifestyle.

I am always thrilled to see the change in skin complexion in many clients after a mere one to two weeks from the difference in their body as they hydrate and follow the PFL. They go from looking pale and tired to fresh and glowing! That says everything to me about how important the principles are in helping our bodies function well.

Caffeine and Dehydration

If you are a heavy caffeine user—defined as taking in 500-600 milligrams or the equivalent of 5-7 cups of coffee daily—the caffeine will act as a diuretic and increase your potential for becoming dehydrated. When you are trying to keep yourself hydrated and give your body the water it needs, this is a counterproductive behavior. All of the research I have gathered on caffeine in order to give you a ball-park range of moderate use falls to 2.5 milligrams per kilogram of body weight. This translates to 150-170 mg for a 140-150 pound woman and 200-225 mg for a 190-200 pound male. Anything over this may have negative impacts on your health, your adrenal glands in particular.

A great population of people are dependent on caffeine for everyday function—a reliance that is often joked about on social media through memes of over-sized coffee mugs and people who look like they haven't slept in days. While sure, this is funny because so many can relate, this is also a great problem. As you learned in the chapter on supplements, too much caffeine is a problem for your adrenal glands, one that you need work to correct if you wish your body to function optimally.

If over-caffeinating is a problem for you, let's take a moment to analyze the chain of events that binds you to a particular behavior. Are you not sleeping enough? Do you need to go to bed earlier? Do you need to prioritize your day so you can create time for essential sleep? Are you simply trying to get by and that's why you're turning to caffeine?

Another form of over-caffeinating is in pre-workouts. Pre-workouts can be beneficial for those who are putting time into effective resistance training to break down muscle tissue. A beneficial pre-workout power has a healthy balance of amino acids with caffeine (usually no more than 100-200 milligrams per serving). However, too many people use pre-workouts as a way to help them get through the day, thanks to the caffeine. We shouldn't be so tired during the day that caffeine is our life-line to get us through.

Soda

It's time to bite the bullet and kick out the soda from your life—there is no need for it! Whether you drink diet or regular soda, habitual consumption of these carbonated beverages may pose eventual health problems. If you typically go for regular soda, you most likely are taking in High Fructose Corn Syrup, a sweetener that has been heavily linked to disease and illness. Even if you opt for the diet soda, you are taking in artificial sweeteners which we discussed in the Triple S chapter.

To make matters worse, no matter which type of soda you choose, it will have carbon dioxide in it—the very chemical gas your body tries to eliminate from your body by exhaling. Although your body always has carbon dioxide in it at any given time, the normal levels are in proportion to the oxygen concentration that is also in your blood. Don't intentionally throw off the harmonious balance in your body by drinking soda.

Chances are that you already know you shouldn't be drinking soda. So why haven't you stopped? Addiction, habit, and lack of correct motivation and goals. Be sure to review Chapters 2 and Chapter 3 as you embark on your journey to quit drinking soda. If you are a heavy soda drinker, you may find that you experience headaches for 3-5 days from the absence of caffeine. You can get through these days by focusing on how much your health will improve by eliminating this habit. You might also slowly wean yourself off by replacing your soda with sparkling water, and then moving to a "bubbles-free" lifestyle.

Dehydration's Consequences

Dehydration can generate both short-term and long-term risks. Do you want to be constipated? Do you want digestive disorders, stomach ulcers, respiratory troubles, fatigue, eczema, acid-alkaline imbalances or urinary infections? Do any of these problems sound like a great thing to have? When I tell you that drinking adequate amounts of water allows the normal functioning of your body and prevents all of these issues, does that motivate you to want to be diligent in your water intake?

Any change you desire to make with your body will require drinking enough water to facilitate that change on a chemical level. H_2O molecules provide your stomach the level of hydration needed to make, maintain, and adjust the quality of the mucus layer that protects the lining of your stomach during the breakdown of protein (this is the only macronutrient that breaks down in the stomach). Water also provides your pancreas with the proper hydration for it to produce pancreatic fluid. This fluid neutralizes acidic chyme which helps with the breakdown of nutrients in your small intestine. Water does a lot of work in transporting and digesting every nutrient you put in your body. Without it, your efforts to change your body will be inhibited, as the main source of moving things around in your body won't be present.

Nearly every organ in your body requires water for proper functioning; check out this list to see the percentage of water that make up these organs:

- Liver: 86%
- Brain: 74%
- Muscle: 76%
- Blood: 83%

- Skin: 70%
- Kidneys: 83%

Practical Application

How many times have you thought you were hungry when, in fact, you were simply thirsty? It's amazing how in control of your appetite you can be when you keep yourself constantly hydrated. If you can prevent those nagging "hungry but actually thirsty" feelings and cravings, how will that improve your ability to follow-through with changing your habits and lifestyle?

It's time to start carrying water with you everywhere you go. The larger your water container, the less frequently you will need to fill it up and the greater tendency you'll have to drink enough when you do drink. I find that carrying a ½-1 gallon of water with me almost everywhere I go does the trick. And I mean everywhere—to work, to the gym, at home, to meetings, and to events.

Now, I know what you're thinking—but Kristy . . . I really don't want to go to the bathroom more!

You're right, the frequency of your restroom visits will probably increase. But going to the bathroom more frequently is something you have to accept—and it's a good thing! The clearer your urine, the better hydrated your body is. Your kidneys adjust their process of filtering and excreting to the amount of water you drink. There is no better measuring tool than to view the color of your urine. Elimination of water helps cleanse your body of toxin buildup and keeps your kidneys functioning properly.

Flavor Enhancers

When drinking this much water, you may feel inclined to have a different and sweeter taste as water can get tasting pretty drab at times. There are many sweeteners on the market like Gatorade mix, Mio, Crystal Lite, etc. I recommend you stay away from these the majority of the time. While preventing large insulin spikes from the lack of sugar content, artificial sweeteners can not only cause you to experience stronger cravings later, but researchers continue to examine presumptive correlations between these sweeteners and disease.

Instead of using artificial sweeteners to enhance your water, try placing freshly cut fruit and/or vegetables at the bottom of a pitcher or container of water. Cucumbers, bell peppers, raspberries, blueberries, oranges, lemons, limes, and apples all provide a very refreshing taste. Not only that, but the drink is very pleasing to the eye. You can also make ice cubes with these delightfully colorful fruit pieces inside. They are a fun way to add some color to clear glasses at a dinner party.

Conclusion

Your body will always need water, and you need to ensure you have enough water in your body to facilitate body composition shifts and health functioning. No matter what your habits have been in the past, you have the power inside you to make positive changes beginning today. Take baby steps to improve and progress. You now know what you need to do—now go apply it.

Make that change!

Pop the Top and Chug-a-Lug!

17

Maintenance
& Miscellaneous Goals

A s the Power Foods Lifestyle is a system of understanding scientific food principles and using verbiage that allows us to get away from the misunderstood concept of calories, we can apply the PFL to nearly any goal or need in eating. As you get more familiar with the representations of peak ranges per macronutrient category, you will be able to adapt your eating habits and keep it simple without micro-managing every little piece of food you put in your mouth.

As a reminder, here are the representations for peak ranges. Take the time to get familiar with the serving size this represents in each of the power foods. Once you do this, you can easily eyeball your portion size.

P: 15-30 grams protein
V: 1-2 cups veggies
C: 20-30 grams carbs
F: 8-12 grams fats

Ranges for lower-case macronutrients:

p: 7.5-15 grams
c: 10-15 grams
f: 4-6 grams

For instance, imagine yourself having a consultation with a Body Buddies coach when you are plateaued and need to make an adjustment to your eating. Your practice of the PFL lingo would make it very easy to understand what we mean if we (hypothetically) recommended only 5 meals, with a PVCF at Meals 1 and 3, a PVF in your meal, and listening to your body for Meals 2 and 4. If you were deficient in energy at these two meals, I'd say have the PVC. If you were feeling a bit hungrier, I'd say have the PVF. I would ask you to gain that intuition of your body in order to understand what your body actually needed, rather than your brain. If you were feeling like a rockstar, I'd encourage you to strip the energy nutrients and have a PV for the in-between meals while still in the fat loss phase of your journey.

If you understood what I just described, you're well on your way to becoming a Power Foods Lifestyle Veteran! These are people who practice this method of eating and thinking for over one year and truly commit to the lifestyle. Now that you understand the PFL is really about principles and how we each choose to apply those principles, realizing no two people are identical in their bodies' needs, we can discuss certain methods for various populations and approaches. For more in-depth discussion of these topics, please listen to the Body Buddies Podcast, or schedule a consultation on *www. body-buddies.com.*

The Power Foods Lifestyle for Maintenance

Once you reach your goal bodyweight, you may wonder what your next goal should be. Where do you go from here? Can you simply eat whatever you want now? No, though you should know those thought processes are normal, as that's how society has programmed you to think. That is a diet mentality, as you have just put an end date on your strategy and approach to eating. Instead, I would like to see you continue onward using the PFL strategies and habit, but consider a few additional perspectives. Keep in mind that the PFL is not just for aesthetics, but for optimal internal health as well. The PFL bridges the gap between these two goals so you can achieve health at the minimum, and aesthetics if you apply the strategies and manipulation in macros that I teach.

Indulgence Meals for Maintenance

One of the adaptations to the PFL you might consider while you are enjoying your newfound body and health is enjoying a few more indulgence meals each week. This might take the form of several different styles, whether it's decreasing your vigilance in turning down the handful of M&Ms sitting in the jar on the counter, or stopping for a pizza on your way home from a stressful day at work. Many PFL veterans quickly find that allowing too many indulgences begins to make a difference in just how "fluffy" they feel. The beautiful part about the PFL is that not much needs to change if you realize you feel this way. You should first, ensure your portion sizes are on point for your balanced PVF, PVC, or PVCF meals, as well as scale back on the number of indulgences you're enjoying.

Guard yourself against the mindset that you've achieved your goal, and you can now have a free-for-all. You have the knowledge to make sure your body is fueled wisely. You also now have a responsibility to keep yourself motivated and focused on that goal for the duration of your life. It is a day-in-day-out decision to choose to eat this way. Though it sounds awesome to say "this gets easier," it doesn't necessarily. While your consistency in making wise decisions gains momentum, I don't know if someone ever hits a point of auto-pilot forever.

I've been following this way of life for over three years at the time I'm writing the second edition of this book. Over this span of time of dialing in and out (between 11 and 20% body fat depending on the time of year, photo shoot dates, and competitions) and everywhere in between numerous times, I have learned there are a few key principles that keep me focused and honed in on where I should be:

1. Weekly goal setting must be a habit. This is the time to pay attention to what needs to change if you're finding yourself making excuses more often, forgetting to food prep, or feeling subpar in any portion of maintaining your new level of health. Review the principles in the chapter on setting goals and make your Sunday evening goals a priority.

2. Understand there are ebbs and flows to life. There will be crazy times in your life full of stress and seemingly impossible times to train and care for your health. Learn to relax just a bit on the rigid approach and simply think in terms of principles. If you're going out to eat, simply think through your principles and do your best.

Don't go crazy—but do not abandon your body's nutritional needs. Typically when a person feels stressed and too busy with life to focus on health, their moods and energy suffer. Stressful times are when you should focus most on fueling yourself and giving yourself the extra physiological advantage. Sleep, nutrition, and exercise are the best coping mechanisms for stressful events, and I encourage you to keep these at the forefront of your mind. Healthy living is actually quite simple when you stop overthinking it.

The Power Foods Lifestyle for Youngsters

Though I do not yet have children at the time I'm writing this book (can't wait for that time in the future!), I have been able to work with many families, parents, and children to improve their nutritional habits.

In the case of overweight children or teenagers, I encourage you to schedule a consultation with myself or one of the Body Buddies coaching team to help direct you in a strategy that will help them specifically with the challenges they face. These have been some of my most treasured times—FaceTiming or Skyping with these children and teenagers when I ask their parents to leave the room and let us talk heart to heart. I would like to share with you some of the principles that we work on in these sessions and hope that you will work to apply them in your own family life little by little.

When discussing nutrition for youngsters, we want to remove much of the rigidity of the original PFL fat loss strategy to focus on fueling them with good foods. Before I discuss that, however, I would like to give you some general overviews of numbers that might help you as you are learning.

The table below sets forth the average daily recommended intake of macronutrients for children ages 4–18, specified by gender. You may notice that the only difference between male and female falls in the slightly higher range for males 14–18 in the protein category, as well as the carbohydrates.

In order to adapt the PFL for these ranges, simply break down the range by 6 (if the child/teenager will be eating all six meals per day.) If not, determine how many meals per day seems more realistic with their school schedule, then divide the daily range by the number of meals. That is the amount of macros in the PVC or PVF meals the child/teenager should have.

I hesitate providing these finite numbers as the data is constantly evolving. Above all, I wish to help facilitate a change to the *awareness of principles*, so let's talk a bit more about how this translates to food. Please, please, please do not use these numbers as a way to micro-manage your children. Again, these numbers are an awareness point as to serving sizes.

As a child's/teenager's body changes as they grow, the hand measurements or estimates of food are generally applicable.

	Male 4-8 yrs.	Female 4-8 yrs.	Male 9-13 yrs.	Female 9-13 yrs.	Male 14-18 yrs.	Female 14-18 yrs.
Protein	20-30 g	20-30 g	30-40 g	30-40 g	40-60 g	40-50 g
Carbs	130 g	130 g	130 g	130 g	130-160 g	130-140 g
Fats	25-35 g	25-35 g	25-35 g	25-35 g	25-35 g	25-35 g

- Protein: 1/2 or the full size of the palm of the hand in thickness and circumference
- Carbohydrates: size of the fingers curled up in a fist from the knuckles down
- Fats: the palm of the hand in a cupped shape for nuts, or the size of the tip of the thumb for oils
- Vegetables: a fist portion size

There will always be exceptions that apply, but this is a good basic guideline. You see, the PFL isn't about perfection; it's about doing better. It's about being aware that there is protein to stabilize the blood sugar throughout the day. It's about ensuring micronutrients are present to repair and help a child's/ teenager's body build and function optimally. These come most fully in the form of vegetables, so having a portion every time they eat is critical. The PFL is easy to implement with youngsters when you take the principles mindset approach, rather than the hard-nosed "eat every 2.5-3 hours and have perfection across the PVC and PVF meal combos."

The Starting Point

Naturally, soda is going to be a pretty big focus as this is a part of mainstream schools with vending machines and the social scenes for developing children and teenagers. Soda is often used by kids and teenagers as a "feel-good" and "stress relief" source. It helps give them a false energy they need to function in an increasingly demanding school environment. Additionally, take a look at their sleep patterns and make goals to get good sleep habits in place. This can naturally eliminate the need for soda simply to cope with fatigue.

Youngsters will function best if they are focusing on drinking their body weight in ounces of water. If a child is overweight, they should be drinking the body weight of a healthy child their age in ounces of water.

Many parents have benefitted from having a "water goal chart" on the kitchen counter where their children can mark the number of cups of water they had each day. As a family, set a goal together about how much water each member of the family should be drinking, then establish a reward for the weekend if everyone hits their goal.

The Next Steps

Children and teens often run out the door to school without eating breakfast. This causes their blood sugar levels to decline and they end up ravenous by the time mid-morning or lunchtime rolls around. Not only will eating breakfast prevent overeating later on in the morning (stay ahead of hunger), but their brains will function more efficiently if they are eating their first meal—a solid PVC (protein-veggie-carb) meal prior to leaving for school. Optimally, this should be within one hour of waking.

Your child should be a part of, if not completely responsible, for packing their lunch each morning or the evening before. Convenience and necessity of feeding many mouths does not allow cafeterias and other fast-grab food franchises to offer high-quality nutritious food that is fresh. A child or teenager following the Power Foods Lifestyle should be taking their food from home to school the majority of the time.

When your child arrives home from school, help them have a healthy and balanced after-school snack (easily referred to as Meal 4 in the PFL). It is okay if something sugary is a part of this meal, but only in addition to the balanced PVC or PVF meal. If the child or teen has after-school activities that prevent them from being at home for a meal, an additional meal should be packed with them as they leave in the morning. The habit of preparing a meal the night before will eliminate the chaos of mornings where everyone seems to be running late.

Planned Motivation is Key

Most people function well when offered incentives and rewards for good behavior, especially children. Planned indulgence meals and other reward systems can be extremely beneficial in making healthy lifestyle changes a reality.

Parents and children should sit down together each Sunday to go over the agenda for the week ahead. Doing so will allow you the opportunity to plan meals, set the indulgence meals to look forward to (i.e. order pizza on Friday night or go out to eat as a family on Saturday night), and also offer other rewards for making strategic choices.

For example: if Joey agrees to pack his balanced PVC or PVCF meals the night each night this week and follows through, mom will grant him amnesty from chores on the weekend. Use the dynamics of your family and the likes/dislikes of the children and teenagers in order to establish rewards that are meaningful to the person changing the behavior.

Parents who use "no sugar" challenges with their children find that the kids keep them on track more than the other way around. Try this for a week, a month, or even several months. Be sure to plan a rewarding finish so all members of the family are incentivized to do their best and follow through with avoiding sugar, soda, or even get as nit-picky as refined oils and processed foods.

Awareness and Education

Youngsters need to be taught to turn over the labels of any food that comes in a package. Teach them where the content of sugar is located (usually toward the bottom of the Nutrition Facts table). Help them notice that if a food has over 5–10 grams of sugar in a portion size, this is not ideal for helping their body function at its best. They will like the taste and enjoy the sugar rush for 5–10 minutes, but then they will experience the cravings that sugar triggers and seems to never turn off.

Help your child learn to identify the source from which their foods come. Teach them which foods come from the earth, and which foods come from a factory. This is what we call processed foods, and will often be filled with additional chemicals that cause less than optimal responses in the body.

A child or teenager may not be able to meet the exact timing that I recommend for the PFL principles. This is okay and is not to be a stressor! Whatever the frequency of meal timing, seek to keep in mind the balance of macronutrients. Keep in mind that the more frequent the meals are, the higher a child or teen's energy levels will be, the greater their nutrient absorption will be, and the greater chance they will have to maintain willpower and ability to biochemically stay away from cravings and overconsumption of food when they do eat.

This is Doable

This is a process, and will require a good support system. Seek to involve friends, family, and even teachers to help support the changes that need to be made. It's not easy—but after 2–3 weeks you'll really start to get it. It will become easy and doable, and soon, they will start seeing changes in their body. They will feel better. Their clothes will start to fit looser, and soon, you will be buying them new clothes (if your child is overweight when starting). It will not happen overnight, so help them be patient and focus on changing their behavior and the results will come. We can change our body by changing our behavior!

Sure, everything is tough at first. There is a learning curve. But most find that after a short two weeks of living a Power Foods Lifestyle that this is easy and they are finding how this truly can be (and does become) their lifestyle. We each want our children to be healthy and happy. Isn't it about time you help your child develop the habits that will make this a reality? I would love to help you accomplish this goal for your family. Please join the private Facebook group Power Foods Lifestyle Champions and gain insights from others living this lifestyle.

The Power Foods Lifestyle for Older Adults

If you are someone who has had your children leave home (or perhaps you never had children and you are around age 50+), chances are your gusto and desire for that "perfect body" has dimmed. That. Is. Just. Fine. The PFL is for you as well. After all, we are discussing nutritional principles that are important for any time of life.

With age comes a need to focus on nutrition in order to give you the highest quality of life possible. Generally, doctors recommend for their older adults a variety of fruits, vegetables, proteins, and whole grains to improve overall health.

Having worked with many people in this demographic, I think the number one obstacle is that you are sick and tired of cooking! For many years you have eaten meals from home, prepared for your children or loved ones, and now that particular phase has passed, you're a bit burnt out. (I'm sure I will be too when I hit that point in my life.) However, the simple fact of preparing your own food versus dining out, which is both a stress-relief and social event, is that you maintain your own control over the nutrients you provide your body.

I recommend to my older adult clients that you try to eat 2/3 of your meals under your own care and jurisdiction, then allow 1/3 of your meals to come from dining out opportunities with friends, family, or your significant other. Keep in mind there are lots of faster ways to prepare foods—we do not need them to all be gourmet dishes. You can fuel your body to preserve and protect your health through small and simple meals.

The second obstacle you face is that you are very set in your ways and have habits that are comfortable. Change is not fun. You will find yourself very skeptical, especially if introducing new foods into your daily food intake. Introduce these changes gradually, as too much at once will repel your desire to invite change into your life. Let's go through a few basic principles to begin introducing, perhaps even one per week.

Meal Timing & Size

Due to lacking the desire to eat as much, you may not eat the full peak range servings of the PVC or PVF meal structure. However, your body will benefit far more if you keep the integrity of the meal combination, and simply reduce the portion size of each food you eat. As you stick to the recommended 2.5-3 hours for snacks and meals, your blood sugar will stay more stable, you will absorb more health-promoting nutrients, and you will have more energy—all of which are outcomes you need if you are wanting to feel as good as possible. Keep in mind that this type of eating will help your cholesterol balance, and keep you looking as vibrant as possible (yep, this includes helping prevent wrinkles, as your skin is a barometer of your overall health!)

Omega 3 Fatty Acids

If you have arthritis, cancer, or heart disease, paying attention to your healthy fats is very important. Healthy fats will also sharpen your mind, and decrease your risk for Alzheimer's disease. You may revisit the chapter on fats to learn which are the best for you, and which to keep in your home. Raw nuts are great to snack on, as well as olives and sardines (if you can stomach them).

Try the strategy of only 1-2 meals you eat as PVC meals and the rest as PVF meals. This is due to the fact that carbs in general can lead to, or promote, inflammation. In some cases, older adults feel best if we completely wipe out the PVC meals and replace them with PVF meals, allowing their bodies to go into more of a ketogenic state where their bodies feed off ketones, as opposed to glucose, for energy and function.

Low Sodium

Many of the Power Foods Lifestyle recipes have sea salt, taco seasoning, or garlic salt recommended for taste. If you have hypertension, it is still okay if you salt your foods lightly. When you are following the PFL recommendations of eating, your sodium intake falls in healthy ranges (around 2,200 mg daily). The problem is when you're eating frozen, processed foods, or dining out frequently. These types of foods come with a much higher sodium content.

Protein Shakes

These drinks will work well for you as they are fast and simple. Not only that, but as you age, your body needs more protein than in your middle-aged years in order to help preserve muscle mass (unless you have diabetes or kidney disease).

I encourage you to make your own shake, and avoid the pre-mixed, highly marketed protein drinks on the market (Ensure®, Slimfast®, etc.). As you look at your nutrition label, check for the sugar content. The same principles apply here as in the regular PFL—let's keep sugar under the 5-10 gram mark, and make sure the protein is falling between 15-30 grams to be what we designate as an excellent source of protein.

Use a high-quality protein powder, which you can find by viewing the products tab of www.body-buddies.com. Be sure to blend into your protein shake some vegetables like kale or spinach, add up to ½ cup of fruit, use a non-dairy milk alternative like almond milk, coconut milk, or cashew milk (all unsweetened), and consider adding 1/4-1/2 c. oats or bran flakes for additional carbohydrates.

The Power Foods Lifestyle for Bulking/Re-Framing

The need or desire to add lean muscle tissue to your frame can help in athletic performance, everyday function and ability, and the reason most people go into a bulk or re-framing period—aesthetic appearance.

I've worked with many men and women to build them in a strategic and healthy way, eliminating the free-for-all mentality and focusing on nutrient-dense overconsumption to promote protein synthesis of new muscle tissue. Due to this experience, I choose to use the word "re-frame" hand-in-hand with "bulk." Most women have demonstrated a fear of the word "bulk" as it denotes a heftier body mass which no woman wants (it's rare that a man displays these feelings as well.) In a society that praises the thin person and applauds those who control their portion sizes to rabbit-sized amounts, it can be a bit daunting to pursue the approach necessary to gain greater results down the road. Understanding this, you need to be psychologically aware of the potential to sabotage your efforts if you fall victim to worrying about how you look and what people think as you are in a bit "fluffier" state.

A great benefit from adding additional muscle tissue to your physique is an increased rate of metabolic burn—a.k.a. you'll burn more calories in a day. Your physique is the shape of your muscles, so when you hear you have a nice physique (most people give me an odd look when they hear me say that), that's referring to the aesthetics of the muscle. You can have a beautiful physique to the astute eye and not be "lean." This means the balance of your muscle groups are well developed and aesthetically proportionate.

How Much Time is Needed?

A true bulk should take around 8-12 months for a sizable difference though you may still see noticeable gains through less time than that. Keep in mind, however, that this evolution of your body takes time (when done naturally without anabolic agents, pro-hormones, or testosterone boosters—banned substances by definition of the World Anti-Doping Agency).

Detrimental to your goal to re-frame your body is not being fully committed to your goal. Keep in mind that you cannot bulk and cut at the same time. Choose your goal—one or the other. You can't do one for a few weeks, then switch to the other expecting to see sizable differences. Your body is a complex system of evolutionary and chemical processes. It needs time and consistency for it to adapt to the new variables you give it. Many programs out there promise more results with less time—gosh, that marketing is so deceptive!

How Much Will You Gain?

If you have a higher than average body fat percentage, you should know that, yes, it's possible to gain muscle while dropping body fat. But once you are at a body fat percentage that is less than average—understanding exceptions apply—you may not gain muscle as you continue to cut. This is due to the fact that you are in a caloric deficit and don't have the nutrients to synthesize new lean muscle tissue. Basically stated, if you're not in a caloric excess, you're not gaining muscle. You might be losing body fat which pulls the skin tighter around the muscles, giving the appearance of bigger muscles, but your muscles did not actually gain size and mass.

You will most likely gain some fat while bulking or re-framing your body. This doesn't have to be sizeable amounts like you see many bodybuilders doing in the off-season, but realize that it's a natural result of giving your body excess nutrients. Eliminate the mentality that you will be shredded while gaining, so you can eliminate the bulking sabotage that happens when you let fear of the fluff set in. This usually manifests itself in unplanned cardio sessions, or eating less than is needed to be in a caloric excess. It is very normal to allow your weight to rise 10-15 lb. above normal for women, and 20-30 lb. above normal for men.

Your body will respond if your strategy is on point, but you must be consistent and determined to continue on with it and maintain it—that's a huge focus here at Body Buddies. We want to maintain the results that we attain through strategic fueling of our bodies. If you don't have the mental discipline to do a true re-framing period, it might be better not to pursue it in a halfway pursuit. You might get confused about your baseline functioning—which is a healthy lifestyle—using the Power Foods Lifestyle.

There are two bulking terms used in mainstream bodybuilding: "clean bulk" and "dirty bulk." A clean bulk is where you eat nutrient-rich foods (in our PFL vernacular that means power foods), or a dirty bulk is where you eat whatever you want in mass quantities. I advocate the "clean" approach, though I don't particularly like that term. As I often say on my podcast, What, did you wash it? Any food—whether nutrient-packed (clean) or empty-calorie foods (dirty)—can be harmful to your health if eaten in too large of quantities. Inner health function is critical as we approach aesthetic goals, and that is why getting the majority of your nutrients and energy through power foods is the more appreciable approach in my humble opinion.

Helpful Key Points

- You might have re-phrasing pants that are a size or two bigger than your maintenance pants. Mentally embrace the fluffier body and remember that this is simply the phase you're in. Enjoy the journey and harbor no negativity toward yourself; focus instead on the changes you're strategically seeking to make.

• Track your progress and the weights you lift for your main exercises in the gym. Assess on a monthly basis with one rep maxes (1RM).

• Stay off the scale. Growth will not be determined by weight. Go off photos instead (monthly).

• Keep cardio in your program for cardiovascular health. Try to do 2-3 sessions of low-intensity cardio for 30 minutes per week. Having a fit and strong cardiovascular system will increase the oxygen uptake into your cells and maximize your training sessions.

• Get a minimum of six hours of sleep a night. If you're serious, and especially if you're a guy, you have more metabolic processes you need to facilitate. Your body recovers and resynthesizes mostly while you sleep. If you're not getting much of it, you're not growing!

• Family, friends, and co-workers might make fun of you for your extra consumption of food and additional layer of fluff, but don't give in to their banter. Know your goal and stick to it.

Adaptation of PFL Principles

1. Take all four of your basic PVC meals and double the carbs. As your peak range is 20-30 grams, then your new range would be 40-60 grams, (making your meals a PVCC). For men taller than 6' and weighing more than 200 lb. you may benefit from 2.5-3x the peak range per carb meal, meaning each PVC meal will have (50-90 grams).

2. Stick to your cup of veggies with every meal, but feel free to do more. The veggies do make you feel full, but it's important to keep your basic nutrition and vitamin sources in your food intake. Many re-framers find that blending their food into a shake makes it easier to get down. Yes, that sounds gross, but when you're trying to pack in that much food each day, sometimes you need all the help you can get. Bulking and re-framing definitely gives you greater appreciation for a cutting mentality!

3. Ensure one of your PVCC meals comes following your training session. Half of the CC should be a power food like quinoa, oats, brown rice, but the other half should be fast-acting sugars like white rice or white rice flour, Pixie Stix, Oreos, Cinnamon Toast Crunch, or a dextrose carbohydrate supplement. This will help your insulin respond more quickly and help absorb the fuel into the cells of the muscles. The half of the carbs that are fast-acting sugars are what I call "sanity carbs." This is a strategic way to get that yummy food you love in your body, but use it at a time that your body will better handle it and optimize the nutrients' properties to get you closer to your goal. This mentality may also be used for a maintenance period, and occasionally can even work when cutting.

4. If you're training at any time other than first thing in the morning, make sure you get a good PVCC for your pre workout meal. If you feel irritated or bloated, it's okay to cut the veggies from that meal and add that portion to a different meal. You might try a PC meal, or a PF meal—as long as you're getting plenty of carbs in the previous 12 hours, you should have enough glycogen to fuel the ATP system for energy in your lifts. Some people feel better on fats before a workout, and some feel better on carbs. Others even feel that a PVCF or a PVCCF pre-workout meal about 1-2 hours prior to the workout lends them tons of energy and the strength they need to lift heavy and with power. If training first thing in the morning, you should be fine with a simple protein shake and carb (PC) as you should have had plenty of carbs in the previous 12 hours. If you can lift on more food in your stomach, however, that would be fine to adapt the meal in that way.

5. Fats should be about 2x the amount of a normal peak range (8-12 g) for a new range of 16-24 grams per meal. These are fine to keep to the end of the day, though they may also be scattered throughout the other meals for additional nutrition and energy. If you're lifting first thing in the morning, you might benefit from additional carbs in the evening with your fats (carb back-loading) and keeping your PVF meals in the afternoon.

Conclusion

I hope that you have learned a lot about just a few of the many ways you may manipulate Power Foods Lifestyle principles for different populations and goals. It's thrilling to discuss goals and approaches with people who speak this lingo—we can get very specific and the client or consumer of information knows exactly how to apply it without being tied to a plan. Thank you for taking the time to educate yourself so you are more informed and can take the reins in controlling your health and reaching your goals!

18

Helpful Tidbits

Time is your greatest asset. If you struggle to manage the hours in your day, you may find yourself struggling to become the person you truly want to be. I don't believe in time management, because we each have the same amount of time each day. Instead, we should work on self-management. Eating healthfully and exercising doesn't have to take a great deal of time, yet I often hear comments from people that they are simply "too busy" for that kind of dedication. Well, Body Buds, I would like to clarify something about these perceived efforts: yes, dedication is an all-day-long event; however, *focusing* constantly on those efforts should not be.

We each have events that comprise many days in our lives—we have jobs, families, hobbies, weddings, break-ups, funerals, birthdays, divorces, births, graduations, vacations, and holidays. Each of these events tends to center around food. Many of our relationships, and the time we share with our loved ones, involves food. How do we live the PFL principles when all of these events will constantly be a part of our lives? Doesn't it seem unrealistic? Many people tend to think so. While this mentality is completely normal as you're looking at it from the outside— I assure you that from where I stand, having lived this lifestyle for nearly three years, it's completely realistic.

A healthy lifestyle should, and will, work in conjunction with your busy and eventful life. Please don't become so fearful of what's involved in living a healthy lifestyle that wise choices seem to be a formidable task and completely impossible in your mind. To help you relax and realize the PFL principles are very possible for you, I would like to share a handful of helpful tidbits to make the process simple.

Tip #1: Cook Simply

Oh the frustration that accompanies appetizing-looking recipes with a lengthy list of ingredients that seem quite foreign and nearly impossible to find. Half of the time, I have no idea what some of the ingredients are—I've never heard of so many odd ingredients! I used to get frustrated and refuse to try the recipe, opting for something familiar and simple. Who has time to find out what that obscure ingredient is, let alone shop for it?

Due to my easily frustrated personality, I choose to cook simple, yet flavorful meals—you'll find these in the Power Foods Lifestyle recipe books. Simplicity is the greatest secret of the PFL, both in ingredients and seasonings. Meals do not need to be elaborate to taste wonderful, and be healthy and satisfying. Cooking simply is how you can and will maintain this lifestyle, especially on a budget and with a family.

When you find a particular meal that works well for you, stick with it! We are all creatures of habit at the root of our existence. One of my favorite "go-to's" is the following:

- 1/2 cup 2% cottage cheese mixed with 1 tsp. dry Ranch powder mix and pepper

- 1 handful of baby carrots

- 12 raw almonds

This is a PVF meal and super easy to throw in a plastic container, along with a plastic spoon, and run out the door to eat on my way. These types of meals that work well for being busy are excellent to use over and over again. Keeping in mind you want a variety of veggies, you might swap out the carrots for ½ cucumber, bell pepper, or ¼ c. green peas. Simplicity will help you pair foods together for quick-grabs instead of relying on recipes all the time. Recipes are wonderful when you have time to prep them, but they are not a must-do to live this lifestyle! I originally created this lifestyle without the recipes—just simply pairing basic foods together for my very busy life at the time. You can do it! Keep it simple, and decide what the best approach for you and your lifestyle will be.

Tip #2: Food Prep

Food prep is the time you should take during your week to prepare the majority of your meals and snacks. This makes it so they are easy to grab when you're in a hurry. Food prep is the secret to success in this lifestyle. Without having pre-cooked meals in containers in my fridge that I can grab and throw in my purse as I head out the door, my natural tendency would be to stop for a hamburger at Wendy's or even go without food—either of these being counter-productive in helping me reach my goals. Not many people have access to a stove, pots and pans, let alone the time to prepare a full meal each time they eat—and with the PFL, you should be eating a minimum of four times per day. That is far too often to be thinking and planning each meal.

When preparing your food requires that much brain power, you will naturally take simpler routes and opt for what is easy and familiar. This can often be the form of sabotage that quickly follows your desires to change your lifestyle. This is a tough learning curve to beat, but you can do it. Every client I have ever worked with will tell you that food prep will make or break you. They know what they're talking about *wink wink.*

Having healthy food ready to go enables you to fuel yourself regularly with the right nutrients your body needs in balance. It takes the guesswork out of eating. It makes your daily list of to-dos possible because you're not wasting time thinking of or preparing food. Food prep—yes it's a noun—is critical to ensure that you reach your goals while continuing to live your life and focus on the things that matter most. Your life doesn't need to revolve around food, and food prep takes the guesswork out of every time your fuel time comes around. It becomes habitual and easy to simply access the meal you prepared, eat it, and move on with your day.

Four parts of your week should be prime time for thinking about food; the rest of your time should be focused on your main priorities of life. Too much thought about your nutrition can cause you to become quite obsessive, though in the beginning this will take a bit more of your attention. Make an effort to only think about your food during these times:

1. While planning your weekly meals and shopping for the groceries to produce these meals.

2. During food prep time.

3. In the morning as you are packing your cooler for the day.

4. Each time you eat a planned meal.

Food prep can be done one to two times each week for the staples if not every meal. To ensure your food is staying as fresh as possible (thus ensuring you actually eat the food you have prepared instead of turning your nose up in disgust and heading for the nearest fast food restaurant), I recommend you have two separate food prep times per week. No matter when you plan to food prep, you need to be sure to schedule it into your weekly plan. Grocery shopping should be done the day before, or the day of, your food prep time. Your food should be as fresh as possible when you begin to prepare it.

An average food prep will take 1-2 hours, depending on the variety of foods you are preparing and the number of recipes (these take longer than simply pairing foods together). Be sure to plan enough time so you are not frustrated by half-cooked food that you must throw into containers and plastic baggies before dashing out the door. If you're spending more than 3 hours in the kitchen, I would encourage you to look at how you're planning your prep. Start with the foods that take the longest, then work your way down. Another tip to keep in mind is what my parents taught me while I was growing up: Chop Chop, Polly Polly! That means, hustle! Stop wasting time and dawdling all over the place. Get the job done!

Begin prepping the food that will take the longest to cook. This will help you to finish your food prep meals around the same time. Be sure to multi-task; while something is in the crockpot or oven, chop your veggies or cook something on the stovetop.

Proteins:
- Grill
- Bake
- Crockpot
- Sauté
- Boil

I recommend not cooking more than 3-4 days' worth of meat as I personally find myself turning up my nose at meat when I do this. Instead, cook 3-4 days' worth of meat, and either marinade the remainder or what you've purchased, or freeze it for an additional prep around Thursday or mid-week of your regularly scheduled eating cycle.

Veggies:
- Raw
- Steamed
- Baggies for Same-Day Microwave Steaming
- Baked
- Sauté

Vegetables can go bad quickly, so I recommend doing an additional grocery store shop mid-week to keep your veggies fresh. Get away from "back-of-the-fridge syndrome," which is where you shove your veggies to the back and never eat them. Preparing your veggies either in a recipe or preparing them in baggies for quick-grabs and fast additions to meals will ensure you do not waste these extremely important foods.

Carbs:

- Crockpot
- Boiled
- Steamed
- Baked

Grain-based carbs can be individually put in baggies. Most complex carbs cook very well in combination with others in a crockpot (legumes, in particular). Try wrapping your yams or red potatoes in tin foil and baking in the oven at 400 degrees Fahrenheit until a fork comes out smoothly (anywhere from 40-60 minutes). Complex carbs taste so much better when cooked with non-MSG chicken bouillon, sea salt, pepper, salsa, and/or additional seasonings. Make your food taste great so you'll enjoy it!

Fats:

- Individual baggies (nuts, olives)

Most healthy fats will be something you add to a cooked meal, unless it's nuts, seeds, olives, avocado, or cheese. Avocado keeps better with the pit left in, sealed in an air-tight plastic baggie (suck all the air out through a small opening before sealing shut). Store oils at room temperature.

At one time or another, I have caught myself having a poor attitude about the time it takes to prep my food each week. There have been weeks, however, when I don't take the time to prep and the week is a disaster in the nutrition department! I have quickly learned that if I want a healthy lifestyle to happen for me, I must invest that time in the kitchen. As my clients learn this as well, they gain greater perspective into taking personal responsibility for the outcome of their health. A good attitude while food prepping will go a long way!

It might be helpful if you embrace educating and motivating yourself further through listening to the Body Buddies podcast, or a motivational YouTube video. You can find the Body Buddies podcast on iTunes or Stitcher Radio and www.body-buddies.com. I record audio segments on every topic under the sun from nutrition to fitness and mental discipline. This is a great resource for you to access free education and empowerment to live a healthier lifestyle.

Take pride in your food prep and snap a pic! Be sure to tag @bodbuds and @powerfoodslifestyle on Instagram, and add the hashtag #PowerFoodsLifestyle or #PFL. Together, we can help others learn how important this lifestyle can be for them and their health.

Tip #3: Keep Plastic Baggies & Storage Containers Handy

These two items will become your best friends as you grow accustomed to food prepping. Storage containers can be expensive, so if you don't find a good deal at your local grocery store, drop by a dollar store and stock up on all you can. You should have a specific area of your kitchen dedicated to storing your containers as you need to have enough to utilize every time you food prep. I have a whole cupboard in my kitchen filled with them, including a shallow box in which I place my lids sideways from smallest to biggest (this is very helpful if you like to be organized like I do).

You will find that certain types of storage containers are better for some foods than others. For instance, a PVC meal fits beautifully in a two-inch deep square container. You wouldn't want to cram all that food into a small little bowl-type container—that would be more suitable for a ½ cup of cottage cheese serving with some oats and berries.

Snack-size plastic baggies are amazing for portioning nuts, protein powder, raw veggies, and fruit. This act of portioning foods seems to always save me from the overconsumption that would happen if I were to simply "grab a handful." Can you relate to this? When we take this mentality to eating, our portions end up being much larger than the actual amount of energy and nutrients our bodies need at that time. Even our power foods should not be over-consumed. Portion size control is a principle that we must always strive to follow. Measuring and being accountable is what makes all the difference in disciplining our minds and allowing our bodies to reach the shape and inner health functioning we desire.

Tip #4: Use Tin Foil for Easy Clean-Up

When baking chicken, fish, turkey, vegetables, potatoes, or just about anything else that goes in the oven, line the cookie sheet or baking dish with tin foil. Lay your food across the tin foil, then choose a different seasoning to keep the variety in your foods. Try using Rosemary, Oregano, Thyme, Garlic Salt, Seasoned Salt (non-MSG), Lemon Pepper, Sea Salt, Pepper, Italian Seasoning, Savory, or other combinations of seasonings listed in the Triple S chapter. Not only does this make for very quick clean-up, but you will find you can prepare many of your foods this way. A typical oven heat for this type of baking is 350-400 degrees Fahrenheit.

Tip #5: Steam your Vegetables or Eat Them Raw

A steamer and large pot in which you can steam a large quantity of vegetables will become your best friend. You can do this so quickly—simply fill the pot up to the steamer line with water, wash and cut up your vegetables, throw the lid on, and turn the heat to high for 20 or so minutes. Be sure to watch the water occasionally so that it doesn't boil dry—I will admit I have occasionally run from the shower to a kitchen full of smoke and a burned-through pan!

I find that pre-steamed vegetables are good for up to around four days in the fridge. That is when I throw another pot on the stove. If you don't have time to steam your vegetables, you can utilize those snack-size baggies to carry around bags of crunchy and nutritionally-intact veggies, or throw them in the microwave for same-day steaming.

Tip #6: Prep your Daily Vitamins

Whether it's a pill capsule container, a small Tupperware, or plastic baggies, distribute your vitamins and supplements by individual days. There are days you just don't have time to open every bottle and pour a capsule into your hand! Try doing this on a weekly/bi-weekly basis to save time. This is also very helpful for traveling.

Tip #7: Utilize Gas Stations

Meals on the road are inevitable—that's why fast food restaurants are so popular! If you have your cooler packed, you can run into a gas station or convenience store, pop your meal in for 30-45 seconds, grab some utensils and you're good to go! This has prevented me on numerous occasions from stopping at my beloved Wendy's or Taco Bell.

Tip #8: Always Plan Ahead

Weddings, funerals, birthdays, you name it . . . eating out will happen. You'll need to find the balance of living a healthy lifestyle while still living your life. Think through the food that might be, or might not be, available.

Make a plan of action. Go online or call ahead to the restaurant to get an idea of their menu. This is a form of visualization that enables you to make a decision based on logic, rather than emotion. Once you get in the environment, surrounded by people you love and the emotion in the air, it can be easy to forget your goals. If you have visualized what you will eat and how you will avoid certain pitfalls, you may find yourself making much wiser choices. Everything in this lifestyle comes down to goal-setting, preparation, and a positive mindset.

Tip #9: Keep your Pantry Stocked

Below are a few pantry items that are useful to keep on hand:

- Olive Oil and Coconut Oil: these are some good basics to have around, though there are several other whole foods oils that are great as well! Replace your vegetable and canola oils with these. Be sure to store in a cool, dry place away from heat (not over the stove).

- Oat or Coconut Flour: this is a light flour that is gluten-free and most stomachs handle it very well. I usually bake with oat or whole wheat flour (which isn't gluten free).

- Unsweetened Applesauce: this is a great substitute for any butter or margarine requirement in a recipe.

Protein Powder: while this is expensive, I have never regretted having several large tubs in my pantry at all times. Estimating one 5 lb. tub of protein powder per month in conjunction with weekly groceries for one, I spend approximately $250 per month as I follow the PFL. Talk about both cost and health-effective! Be sure to check out my current protein powder recommendations by visiting www.body-buddies.com.

Tip #10: Stick to PFL principles when Dining Out

Going out to eat can often seem very scary and something we don't like to do when we are working hard toward reaching our goal. But with the following principles, you will be armed to make the best choice for you, no matter the restaurant. Well, I suppose we should qualify that, there will definitely be some restaurants where there are no healthy options. But a typical American-style family restaurant will give you what you need.

1. Order a salad or steamed vegetables. The salad can have any kinds of fresh, raw veggies—but no cheese, no nuts, nothing added to it. Choose to skip the dressing and ask for a side of salsa or some lemons or limes that you can squeeze over the

top. You can often swap a side for the steamed veggies. Ask specifically that they not be cooked in any oil (or they will!). I like to lie a lot (ha ha) and say that my body has very adverse reactions to oil, so please be very careful with my food and tell the chef. If you ask what type of oil they use, prepare yourself not to be surprised when it's canola, soybean, or vegetable oil—the very oils that are linked to high cholesterol.

2. Lean protein. Fish. Chicken breast. Sirloin. Shoot for 4-6 ounces. Make sure it's not dressed in any sauces or cooked in oils. Once again, ask specifically that it not be.

3. Choose Carbs or Fats, depending on the menu availability. Just don't choose both—you'll still get residual energy nutrients from whichever you choose. You could choose a 3-oz. yam (probably need to cut it because they'll serve you one too large), or a slice of fresh wheat bread. (Skip out on the appetizer breads as they're usually all refined breads with a high glycemic index.) Any kind of beans (1/2 c.-- stick to this portion usually) or whole wheat noodles (no dressing or sauces—it will be purely fat and carbs) or go the Fats route by asking for 1/2 an avocado. That's usually the go-to, unless you keep a baggie of nuts in your pocket or purse.

4. Drink water. Water. Water. Water. It helps, especially when you're surrounded with yummy food. I usually joke with my server and inform him or her that I'll need a large pitcher, or they will be pouring water for me all night!

5. Though it's tempting and takes mental fortitude, skip out on dessert. Can you have a bite? Yes. Help your company feel that you are not weird. One bite won't hurt you (unless you're one of my contest prep athletes—this might be problematic in actuality). Comment on the flavor, the appeal, etc. Say that you don't have the appetite for a full dessert on your own.

6. Any negative commentary (which can easily happen when one person orders extremely healthy foods) can be negated by joking that you'll get a tummy ache if you don't, or that you'll be sick tomorrow—something like that. I usually choose the "doesn't work with my body" route instead of the "I'm eating healthy" route. It just sits better with others and they can't argue their bias toward how you look or what you should be doing. People need to mind their own business, but they rarely do. Accept it, and don't let it affect you. Be your best version of you.

Tip #11: Establish your baseline mode of functioning

At the end of the day, this lifestyle can be tough to manage when you have catastrophic events, life stress, travel, and overloaded schedules that take every ounce of your mental capability to configure. I understand that, and work with clients to establish their baseline mode of functioning. This should be your default zone—the minimum of what you expect of yourself when functioning in high-stress situations with little time or ability to dedicate to your health. Some of the basics that we work together to establish (realizing that you need to adopt your own personal standard and stick to it) include the following:

- At the minimum...I will do five minutes of jumping jacks, sit-ups, pushups, and other bodyweight exercise before going to bed.
- At the minimum...I will drink water over other beverages.
- At the minimum...I will not drown my food in sauces, syrups, and dressings.
- At the minimum...I will try to have a serving of veggies several times a day.
- At the minimum...I will limit myself to one sweet treat each day.
- At the minimum...I will be aware of getting protein at my main meals.

Don't those sound realistic? That's because we have to have our fallback principles—the very purpose of the PFL is to get us doing better, making wiser choices based on nutritional science. We are all human beings and have hectic lives, but we can focus on some of the basic, simpler principles until we have the stability and structure in our day to apply more strategy and get greater results.

Conclusion

I hope you find these tidbits to be helpful as you make way on your journey toward a healthier lifestyle. These tidbits should give you ideas of how to adapt things in your own life and see that the Power Foods Lifestyle is very possible to live when you prepare. It's not initially easy—a healthy lifestyle is not a passive lifestyle. Your health and reaching your goals require an alert mind that is willing to plan and prepare. Committing to this lifestyle is the best thing you can do for your health. You are stronger than you know! You are more capable than you know! The sky is the limit—your mind is the only thing stopping you! All things are possible for those who believe in themselves and trust in God. Be bold! Be brave! Be relentless! Be hungry for change!

"Strategy without tactics is the slowest route to victory."
—*Sun Tzu*

"Strategy is a system of expedients; it is more than a mere scholarly discipline. It is the translation of knowledge to practical life, the improvement of the original leading thought in accordance with continuously changing situations."
—*Helmuth von Moitke the Elder*

19
Pursuit of Perfection

A fter my grandparents passed away during my college years, I ended up living in their home for six months until it was sold. I initially enjoyed living alone during that time of a chaotic college student schedule, but the seemingly peaceful environment quickly began to foster self-punishment. I began using the situation of solitude and privacy as a way to inflict painful "motivation" to improve my perceived physical imperfections. On the inside of every kitchen cupboard I pasted a magazine cutout of a very attractive, lean model. On the walls of nearly every room in my home, I posted sayings like these:

"If you think you're fat, fix it."
"Stop being a wuss and suck it up. Just do it."
"Only lazy people don't achieve their goals."

I even had a little song I made myself sing before bed every night. I will never forget it because of how much I forced these words through my lips:

A little bit thinner
A little bit tighter
Come on, Kristy, you can be a fighter!
Don't give up
Stay on track
You're new body's in the sack!

Though you might argue the words are positive, the way I treated myself day to day was not. Negativity filled the space around me. The images of airbrushed, perfect women clipped from magazines made me realize just how flawed and imperfect I was by comparison. Every time I looked in the mirror (which was a frequent occurrence, given that this period in my life was characterized by daily dance training sessions of 4+ hours wherein I sported tight-fitting and revealing clothing) my self-esteem eroded further.

Despite my logical awareness that perfection was an unattainable myth, I found myself constantly striving to achieve it. Audience members and fellow dancers told me how great I looked onstage and what a beautiful body I had. Regardless of how often I heard these compliments, I remained ashamed of my figure and therefore couldn't acknowledge kind words with sincere gratitude.

What I didn't realize at the time is that achieving the aesthetically improved figure I desired was very possible, though it should have been a secondary, rather than primary goal. At the time, I didn't have the tools or resources to enhance my appearance and health and, as my aimless attempts proved fruitless, this lack of knowledge and proper application resulted in self-loathing.

Embracing the New Me

I am happy to say that now, over nine years later, I no longer perceive myself as a perfectionist. I definitely hold a high standard for myself, but in a healthy and happy way. I can honestly tell you I love my body.

I am now able to maintain the aesthetically improved figure for which I longed and worked. I now accept different phases of my training—from cut and ripped, to softer and fuller. (Notice how I don't say fatter or skinnier?) I have the tools, education, and experience in dialing my body in and out of what the public views as a "rockin' bod" over 12 times, and will probably be doing so, experimenting and having fun with it, for the rest of my life. When others might think I've become weak with a softer frame during certain months of the year, I embrace and accept where my body is because I am choosing to put my body there. I control my behavior and the outcome of my body's look and health through modification of the principles I teach to people like you every single day.

More important than the change in my physical appearance, however, have been the dramatic increases in my levels of health and happiness on a psychological and emotional level. Through my experiences, I have learned—and continue to learn—a great deal. I'd like to share with you the most influential principle that I discovered during my struggles in the hopes that you will grasp its truthfulness and apply it in your own life.

If I had merely focused on changing my physical appearance and hadn't worked as earnestly on changing my cognitive patterns and the triggers that caused my unhealthy behaviors, my results would be far different and far less effective. Sure, I could still reach the physical appearance I wanted, but my mind would still be trapped in the cycle of self-loathing and never being "good enough."

I have since coached many people to their dream body goal. I give them tools and education to help them with the inner transformation as well, but it's up to each person to utilize those tools. It's an unfortunate event when I hear from a client, "Kristy, I have my dream body, but why do I still feel empty inside?" This sincere question from the avid pursuer of change breaks my heart as something inside them was not yet ready for the change.

Aesthetic Improvement is Empty without Inner Improvement

As you seek to improve your physical appearance and health through the Power Foods Lifestyle principles and strategies, it is extremely important that you also focus on changing from the inside out. This takes a focus of reprogramming your mind to view life positively through a lens of optimism. You can start by encouraging yourself, accepting yourself, forgiving yourself, and lifting yourself up with positive thoughts.

I believe it is a noble goal to have both the outer and inner parts of ourselves match each other in their levels of control, discipline, and self-respect. I find that many of the people I work with start to see physical changes in their body only as they apply the cognitive strategies that are essential for success. Our physical bodies simply exemplify our inner thoughts and feelings.

Is there such a thing as perfection? Certainly not in this life. Despite this reality, many individuals—my former self included (she feels like such a distant person now)—often get caught up in subconsciously or consciously trying to achieve the unattainable, then beating ourselves up for failing to reach it. It's a no-win situation. We can't attain perfection, yet we become angry, bitter, and miserable when we don't achieve it.

Then we have the other side of the coin. Does the lack of achieving perfection mean we should accept mediocrity—or even less than that—and tailspin into unhealthy habits? Is this movement for self-love and self-acceptance the opportunity to sit back and say "anything goes" as long as you love yourself?

The answer to both of these questions is *no*. We should neither be placated by laziness nor obsessiveness. We should continue trying to improve ourselves. That's it. End of story. Every day is simply about improvement and progression.

Decrease the Number of Mistakes

I'd like to tell you about my world of dance. As a member of this artistic community, reality can be very harsh. Coaches and teachers often push for their dancers to achieve perfection. I have been on both sides of the spectrum in that regard—on the receiving end as a student of dance, and the giving end as a coach and teacher.

I was grateful to learn an important principle, one that I was able to drill into the minds of my girls. Now when I coach and teach (having taught hundreds of dancers over the years), I always try to get across one crucial point, even requiring my students to repeat the following phrase after me:

Perfection is not my goal.
My goal is to decrease my number of mistakes.

This principle applies directly to the context of your health and body shape. You shouldn't be striving for perfection in eating and exercise habits. Instead, you should be looking for areas in which to do a little better and be a little stronger. This is true especially when we have a farther way to go in our journey toward health. Do you have 50+ pounds to lose? Does it seem impossible and out of reach? It's not. I promise you that it isn't. Change is about baby steps and making one improvement or better choice at a time. If you fail to approach your health from this mindset, you may easily become overwhelmed and feel inclined to throw out every effort, returning to your familiar and comfortable habits.

Baby steps. Progress. Decreasing the laziness or lack of effort. That is what you can—and should—expect of yourself.

High Aesthetic Standards

So what if you have a goal to look better than "average?" Is that goal filled with vanity and pride? Is it okay to strive for a more elite level of aesthetics? I think the answer to this question can only be found within yourself and depends on your personal motivation. Finding your true motivation requires looking deep inside yourself and asking difficult questions with enough confidence to answer honestly.

As I coach both male and female athletes who compete in bodybuilding competitions, I truly do love and support the art of disciplining oneself to a competitive level. The science of the body fascinates me and how control of different variables in nutrition and exercise elicit different responses. However, I put every effort into reminding myself and my clients why we do what we do.

Mastering oneself must be for the sake of discipline and progress. While competition implies judgment, the goal should never be to look "better than others." That is a very childish reason to try to improve. Instead, the goal should be to improve upon oneself. If you are simply a person with an insatiable drive to improve yourself and to conquer obstacles, then I believe it's wonderful to push yourself to extreme levels, as long as you do it with physical and mental health at the forefront of your efforts, and seek to keep your life in balance.

Define "Extreme"

"Perfect is the enemy of good." This quote reminds me that it's easy to lose sight of all the things you are temporarily sacrificing in your pursuit to better yourself. Whether it be a relationship, peace of mind, time with your loved ones, or your overall demeanor, pushing yourself will come at a price. What will you give up for your goal? What preparations and mental checks must you implement to keep balance? Be sure to keep your goals in perspective and your life will be much more fruitful and blessed.

In my former life, I did just about everything wrong in my extreme efforts to reach an unrealistic level of perfection. I hope that others do not push themselves to the extent that I did. The term "extreme" is subjective, a word that has a definition largely dependent on your individual background, experience, and lifestyle. To one person, a very regimented diet may not be extreme at all, while to another, such a nutritional plan may be the most cruel, torturous activity they have ever encountered.

Conclusion

Establish your own definition of "extreme," then work to avoid crossing that line. In the end, stay true to your personal definition. The opinions of others really don't matter in the end so long as your goals result in your improved health. Do your best. Be your best. Just don't try to be perfect.

20

Conclusion

Y ou will do exactly that which you train you mind to do. You know all you need to know. You can begin applying principles of the Power Foods Lifestyle one by one, or jump right in and do it all at once. You have a gift—the ability to think for yourself. You get to choose what you do on a daily basis. You get to decide what you want to become. You get to determine the habits and patterns you integrate into your life on a daily basis.

Throw your fear of failing out the window. It doesn't matter how many diets haven't worked for you. This isn't a diet. This is a lifestyle. This is a way of living that is based on scientifically proven principles. This is a lifestyle that you can easily maintain and enjoy your entire life as you choose which principles are those you should incorporate in your life.

Failure is not an option—the definition of failure is when you stop trying. As long as you are making baby steps forward, you are on the right track. Even if you happen to take a huge step backward, that's okay! Begin your baby steps forward again. Get back up. Brush yourself off.

Keep your eye on the never-ending goal of doing your best each day. I know you will continue trying. Perfection is not the goal. The only goal is to decrease the number of things you know you could be doing better.

I believe in you. Let's make this happen for you. A healthy lifestyle.

Yes, you deserve it.
Yes, you're worth it.
Yes, you can do this.

Love your bud,

Kristy Jo

P.S. Please be sure to check out the many resources I have created and share via my mind and body transformation company, Body Buddies. I'm sure you know someone who may benefit from learning these simple principles. I hope you will share this information with them.

P.S.S. I hope you will email me with your story of improvement, change, and hope. I value every positive email I receive. You may reach me at kristyjo@body-buddies.com.

Website: www.body-buddies.com
Podcast: "Body Buddies" on iTunes and Stitcher Radio
Facebook: www.facebook.com/bodbuds
Instagram: @bodbuds, @powerfoodslifestyle, @teambodbeasts, @PFL2go
YouTube: www.youtube.com/bodbuds

The Power Foods Lifestyle™

Power Foods List

Protein

- Chicken Breast/Tenders
- Cottage Cheese (2% fat)
- Egg Whites**
- Elk
- Ground Turkey (>94% fat)
- Halibut
- Lean Ground Beef (>90% fat)
- Lean Pork
- Lean Sirloin Steak
- Mahi Mahi
- Orange Roughy

- Plain Greek Yogurt (2% fat)
- Protein Powder
- Red Snapper
- Salmon
- Shrimp
- Swai Filet
- Tilapia
- Tofu
- Tuna (packed in water)
- Turkey Breast (nitrate-free deli meat)

Fats

- Almond Butter
- Almond/Cashew Milk (unsweetened)
- Almond Flour
- Avocado
- Bacon
- Butter
- Cheese
- Chia Seeds
- Coconut
- Cream Cheese
- Egg Yolks

- Flax Seeds
- Hummus
- Nuts (Almonds/Brazil/Cashews/ Pecans/Walnuts/Peanuts)
- Oil (100% extra virgin Olive Oil/ Coconut/Flax Seed/Avocado/ Macadamia)
- Peanut Butter
- Pecans
- Pumpkin Seeds
- Olives

Veggies

- Arugula
- Asparagus
- Bell Pepper
- Broccoli
- Brussels sprouts
- Carrots
- Cauliflower
- Celery
- Collard Greens
- Cucumber
- Edamame
- Egg Plant
- Green Beans
- Jicama
- Kale
- Mushrooms
- Mustard Greens
- Romaine Lettuce
- Spaghetti Squash
- Spinach
- Summer Squash
- Sweet Peppers
- Tomatoes
- Zucchini

Carbohydrates

- Apples
- Bananas
- Beans (Black/Kidney/Lima/Navy/Pinto)
- Blueberries
- Bran Flakes
- Bread/Tortilla (Whole Wheat/Rye/Corn)
- Chickpeas
- Couscous
- Ezekiel Bread/Cereal (original)
- Flour (Barley/Oat/Coconut/Wheat)
- Grapefruit
- Grapenuts®
- Lentils
- Oats
- Oranges
- Pumpkin
- Quinoa
- Raspberries
- Red Potatoes
- Rice (Long-grained Brown, Basmati)
- Strawberries
- Whole Wheat Pasta
- Yams

Peak Range Exchanges for Macronutrients

Veggies are all exchanged at 1-2 cups—mix and match as desired

Protein (15-30g)

- 3-5 oz. Chicken Breast/Tenders
- ½-1 c. Cottage Cheese (2% fat)
- 4-8 Egg Whites**
- 3-5 oz. Elk
- 3-5 oz. Ground Turkey (>94% fat)
- 3-5 oz. Halibut
- 3-5 oz. Lean Ground Beef (>90% fat)
- 3-5 oz. Lean Pork
- 3-5 oz. Lean Sirloin Steak
- 3-5 oz. Mahi Mahi
- 3-5 oz. Orange Roughy
- 1/2 -1 ¼ c. Plain Greek Yogurt (2%)
- Protein Powder (Check label)
- 3-5 oz. Red Snapper
- 3-5 oz. Salmon
- 3-5 oz. Shrimp
- 3-5 oz. Swai Filet
- 3-5 oz. Tilapia
- 6-12 oz. Tofu
- 3-5 oz. Tuna (packed in water)
- 3-5 oz. Turkey Breast (nitrate-free deli meat)

Carbohydrates (20-30g)

- 1 med (220 g) Apples*
- 1 med (120 g) Bananas*
- 1/2 -3/4 c. Beans (Black/Kidney/Lima/Navy/Pinto)
- 1-1.5 c. Blueberries*
- 1/2 -1 c. Bran Flakes (check labels)
- Bread/Tortilla (Whole Wheat/Rye/Corn)
- 1/8-1/4 c. Chickpeas
- ½-3/4 c. Couscous
- (check label) Ezekiel Bread/Cereal
- (check label) Flour (Barley/Oat/Coconut/Wheat)
- 1 med. (250 g) Grapefruit*
- ¼-1/3 c. Grapenuts®
- ½-3/4 c. Lentils
- 1/3-1/2 c. Oats
- 1 med. (9 oz.) Oranges*
- 1/3-1/2 c. Pumpkin
- ½-1 c. cooked Quinoa
- 1-1.5 c. Raspberries*
- 3-5 oz. Red Potatoes
- ½-3/4 c. cooked Rice (Long-grained Brown, Basmati)
- 10-15 large Strawberries*
- ½ -3/4 c. cooked Whole Wheat Pasta
- 2-4 oz. Yams

Fats (8-12g)

- 1 Tbsp. Almond Butter
- 3c. Almond/Cashew Milk (unsweetened)
- 2-3 Tbsp. Almond Flour
- 2-3 oz. Avocado
- 1-2 strips Bacon
- ½-1 Tbsp. Butter
- ½-3/4 c. shredded Cheese
- 1 oz. Chia Seeds
- 3 Tbsp. Coconut
- 1 oz. Cream Cheese
- 2 Egg Yolks
- 3 Tbsp. Flax Seeds
- ¼ c. Hummus
- 2 Tbsp. Nuts (Almonds/Brazil/ Cashews/Pecans/Walnuts/Peanuts)
- 2-3 tsp. Oil (100% extra virgin Olive Oil/Coconut/FlaxSeed/Avocado/ Macadamia)
- 1 Tbsp. Peanut Butter
- 2 Tbsp. Pecans
- ½-1 oz. Pumpkin Seeds
- 10-20 large Olives

Be careful on fruits—I recommend sticking to the 'c' rather than the 'C' serving due to the fructose and having 1/3-1/2 the exchange listed in this column if looking to lose body fat

You can easily look up the nutrition facts in any food using myfitnesspal.com or caloriecount.com, both of which have apps for your smart phone. As you get used to the ball park ranges of foods, this lifestyle becomes very easy to pair your nutrients and think critically about balancing your foods.